THE ALKALINE LIFE

THE
ALKALINE
LIFE

New Science to Rebalance Your Body,
Reverse Aging, and Prevent Disease

ROSS BRIDGEFORD

HAY HOUSE, INC.
Carlsbad, California • New York City
London • Sydney • New Delhi

Copyright © 2024 by Ross Bridgeford

Published in the United States by: Hay House, Inc.: www.hayhouse.com®
Published in Australia by: Hay House Australia Pty. Ltd.: www.hayhouse.com.au
Published in the United Kingdom by: Hay House UK, Ltd.: www.hayhouse.co.uk
Published in India by: Hay House Publishers India: www.hayhouse.co.in

Cover design: Julie Davison
Interior design and composition: Greg Johnson/Textbook Perfect
Indexer: Shapiro Indexing Services

Cataloging-in-Publication Data is on file at the Library of Congress

Tradepaper ISBN: 978-1-4019-7578-4
E-book ISBN: 978-1-4019-7579-1
Audiobook ISBN: 978-1-4019-7580-7

10 9 8 7 6 5 4 3 2 1
First Edition, January 2024

Printed in the United States of America

This product uses papers sourced from responsibly managed forests. For more information, see www.hayhouse.com.

To Tania, Leo, Joe, and Kai

Contents

Introduction

My first book, *The Alkaline Reset Cleanse*, was all about the kick start. It gave you the blueprint for the most sensational reboot for your body and to get you moving with six months' worth of results in just 21 days.

And I've been so thrilled to hear the results that the folks who followed my cleanse have achieved. It's one of my biggest accomplishments, and the e-mails I receive daily from people fill me with so much joy and positivity. It has honestly been one of the most incredible things to experience during these last few challenging years.

But while that is the start, the book you have in your hands now is the complete plan. This is how to make it happen, and make it stick, *for life*.

And this is something I've dedicated my life to. A lot has changed since 2003, when in earnest, I coded my first web page to share my alkaline thoughts and ideas (yes, pre-Facebook, pre-blogging, pre-YouTube. It was more Ask Jeeves than TikTok). I remember my first article, my first subscriber, and the first sale of my Alkaline Diet Course 1.0 like it was yesterday—but, wow, things were different then.

Back then my passion was strong. I was a 23-year-old boy with a big idea! I was writing and researching, and my entire business plan was to travel to Tony Robbins events to hand out my little flyers (until they kicked me off-site*).

---

* Tony and I patched things up later.

My life has changed somewhat dramatically since then. I now have three busy boys, am living on a different continent, and have a thriving, ever-evolving business that I love. And holy smokes, life is busy.

Frankly, those days as a young man with a dream and a backpack full of homemade flyers seemed like a much simpler time. But the lessons I've learned in my own life about how to juggle and *prioritize* health while maintaining a relentlessly busy schedule have been invaluable.

I've had serious slipups, just like everyone else—periods when I almost lost myself. But every experience taught me more valuable lessons that have made me a far better coach. I understand what it's like to feel like you can't possibly fit another thing in your life, but you still need to find time for your health.

Every lesson I've learned, alongside my experience of coaching thousands of people to health within *their* busy, hectic lives, has gone into this book.

TRUST

My message has remained consistent over these 20 years, and it really comes down to *trusting your body.* Trust that your body knows what to do and how to do it. Trust that your body knows how to heal, rebalance, rebuild, and thrive.

This has never been more important. And as we're on the cusp of the AI revolution (who knows what this will look like by the time you're reading this book), it's harder than ever to know whom or what to trust.

In a day and age when a hot-looking 21-year-old can open an Instagram account and start selling health advice and supplements overnight, when "influencers" are saying that kale is bad for us (then spinach is bad for us, then legumes, then broccoli—what's next? Air?), it can be a little exhausting.

And so, I want to earn this trust with you.

If you read *The Alkaline Reset Cleanse,* you know I'm *heavily* into the studies and the data, and you'll see this again in this book.

Everything I teach is verified in the literature. I will not tell you to do something without the evidence. And this is verified with my practical experience and the results I see with students in my Alkaline Life Club. These absolute rock stars are living alkaline and getting results day in, day out, and you will see many of their stories over the next few pages.

Their results with challenges such as cancer, heart disease, osteoporosis, fibromyalgia, rheumatoid arthritis, chronic fatigue, acid reflux, brain tumors, fatty liver, and more are amazing. But more amazing is the difference it has made in their quality of life to get out of pain and fatigue and into their true health and energy. Being able to follow their passions, spend quality time with loved ones, pursue dreams, and experience more fulfillment—this is what it's really all about.

LIFE (AND FOOD) IS ABOUT ENJOYMENT AND FUN

In my 20 or so years of helping people, the one constant that I continue to double down on is that any health plan must be *achievable, realistic, fun, and delicious*.

I feel like over those almost two decades, I've gotten pretty good at delivering on this, and I've continued to try to improve my coaching. What you have in your hands right now is the very best step-by-step coaching to living a sustainable and doable Alkaline Life.

In just the last three or four years, I've leaned into the psychology of behavior change, building beneficial habits that stick, and breaking the habits that don't serve us. You will see all this woven throughout the book. It might not always be obvious, but there's a *ton* of research into best-practice habit forming inside these pages. It's all designed to make living alkaline as easy and enjoyable as possible.

Because life is meant to be enjoyed! We are meant to live with smiles on our faces.

What you will *not* find in this book is a hard-core "diet." You will not be told to give everything up, do it all at once, push through pain and cravings, or suck it up and rely on your willpower. That is not living, and frankly, it does not work.

I really mean this. Don't cut anything out. Just focus on the good.

Again, life is meant to be enjoyed. Food can be a source of this enjoyment. I never want you to lose that or feel guilt around it. Food can be a wonderful source of pleasure, connection, and joy. But alongside this, the biggest smile will come from feeling energy, vitality, and strength and the level of connection you feel with your true self when your health is abundant.

When you focus on the good, it *feels* so easy. And when it feels easy, you enjoy it; you stick to it. And when you stick to it, you get results.

But isn't getting started supposed to be the hardest part?

Not with me. Not with the plan you have in this book. My first, single focus for you is to get results quickly.

Results bring confidence. Confidence brings motivation. Motivation brings momentum. And momentum brings results.

You'll avoid overwhelm, stress, cravings, pressure, pain, or any need for willpower. As you'll discover on page 186, willpower is a myth anyway. It doesn't work. So let's not rely on it. Let's make living alkaline so fun, and so delicious, and so easy, you naturally just *want* to do it, stick to it, and look forward to it.

HERE'S HOW THIS WILL WORK

In Part I, I give you the Foundations of the Alkaline Life, where you'll learn what it means to "live alkaline" and what this looks like in the real world. Importantly, I'll bust the ridiculous myths and misunderstandings and show you the science (don't worry, I keep it light!) around how and why the body needs this alkaline balance. You'll learn how to create the biggest impact on your health as quickly as possible, with the least amount of hard work and stress.

I will also show you what happens when you fall out of balance and the impacts this has on your health and longevity. You'll learn the foundational steps of the Alkaline Life, including the foods to focus on and avoid, and the practical steps of getting set up and started.

Then in Part II, we move into The Alkaline Life and Your Goals, covering the most common health challenges and the link between these and acidity. I'll show you the most powerful, laser-focused steps for you to add to your Alkaline Life Plan for *your* individual goals. We cover weight, energy, cancer, atherosclerosis, stronger bones, digestion, autoimmune conditions, and more. You'll have an understanding like never before, which will motivate and inspire you to step into Part III . . . the Alkaline Life Plan!

Part III is the day-by-day, step-by-step breakdown of effortlessly living the Alkaline Life. It is 14 delicious, varied, immensely enjoyable days of alkaline living. You'll have the complete blueprint, along with shopping lists, recipes, advice, and encouragement to see you through. I've covered everything, so you can rapidly get results and build that confidence and momentum without any overwhelm, stress, cravings, hard work, or willpower needed. You can use this baseline plan as the foundation for a lifetime of alkaline living.

The Alkaline Life is natural, whole-food based, nourishing, flexible, and proven. It is intuitive, it makes sense, and it puts you in alignment with your body. You feel in tune. And that feels wonderful. This is all about loving and nourishing your body, and it will repay you tenfold. I can't wait to hear your story and the results you achieve with the simple steps in this book.

So, let's do this!

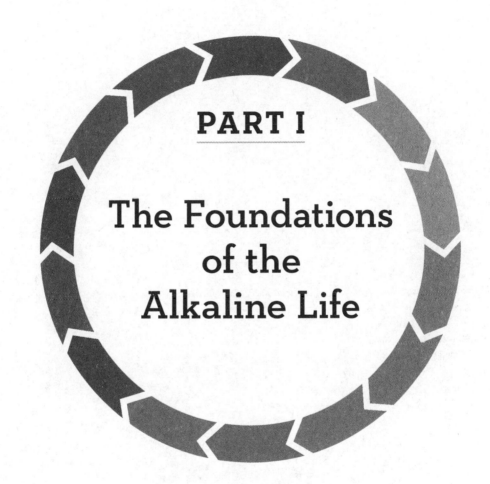

PART I

The Foundations of the Alkaline Life

CHAPTER 1

What *Is* the Alkaline Life?

Your body craves alkaline balance. This is indisputably proven in scientific literature. Study after study shows us that maintaining the correct pH throughout the organs, cells, and fluids in your body is important to every system and process required to keep you healthy and thriving. From your hormonal balance to your digestion, your immune system to your cognitive health, your body works tirelessly to be in pH balance all day, every day.

Yet our modern diet and lifestyle is almost the exact opposite of what the body needs to maintain our delicate pH balance. The way many of us eat today puts the body under constant stress. The modern diet of fast food, convenience food, processed food, sugar, gluten, chemicals, and preservatives drives our pH down, day in and day out, forcing the body to work to bring the pH back to where it needs to be.

And maintaining our pH balance is not just important; it is *essential*. Eating and drinking in a way that puts the body into an acidic state, known as *diet-induced acidosis*, has been proven to dramatically increase the risk of cancer,[1] atherosclerotic disease,[2] neurodegenerative disease,[3] and type 2 diabetes.[4] These are by far the biggest killers in the developed world.[5]

This type of diet has also been proven to increase the likelihood of the "foundational" diseases of autoimmune disease, fatty liver disease, chronic kidney disease, osteoporosis, chronic fatigue, fibromyalgia, adrenal fatigue, irritable bowel syndrome, and more. In fact, the risk of all-cause mortality (dying from anything!) goes up dramatically.[6, 7, 8]

But when we give our body the nutrients it needs to easily maintain our pH balance, everything changes. Abundant health becomes effortless. Your vitality and energy skyrocket, and your risk of disease dramatically lowers. You look and feel amazing.

This is the Alkaline *Life*.

A SIMPLE SOLUTION

Your body, cardiovascular system, endocrine system, aging, immunity, digestion, and brain are all very complex. Sickness and disease are incredibly complex. And the science behind alkaline balance is incredibly complex too.

But the *solution* to living a vibrant, healthy, energized, alkaline life is simple.

The core premise is this: *your only job is to give the body the tools it needs to thrive.*

You don't have to stress or worry about anything else. I repeat, you simply give the body the tools it needs to thrive.

And Mother Nature has provided us with these tools. The wonderful, abundant nutrients in nature are all we need. The vitamins, minerals, antioxidants, plants, water, sunlight, and air are all there for us in abundance. When you combine the power of Mother Nature with the awesome ability of your body to heal and thrive, magic happens.

We will dive into exactly what these nutrients are as we progress forward, but the common thread is that they are:

- alkaline forming
- antioxidant rich
- anti-inflammatory

Foods with these nutrients are abundant in nature. And while some recommended foods are more alkaline than others, and some are more anti-inflammatory, they all contribute to the goal of providing balance in the body.

BALANCE IS ESSENTIAL

The biggest mistake I see with most diet approaches today is that they demand so much change and perfection from day one.

This does not work for 99 percent of people.

It's essential to start small and take little steps day by day, building one success on top of the last. When we try to change everything at once, our brain actively scans for the things we've deprived it of. We make it too hard for ourselves—with too many rules, too much stress, too much pressure. And it's crazy to think, when we decide to change everything at once, that we'll become experts in everything at once. It leaves us exposed to making mistakes and being underprepared, as well as susceptible to lapses in willpower.

If you're the sort of person who likes to highlight things in books, this is a good one for you: *most people wildly underestimate the benefits they can gain by consistently practicing just a small number of positive actions.*

In other words, you can get huge results from tiny changes.

This is central to my coaching. It's so important. To start seeing dramatic progress toward your goals, you do *not* need to change everything. You just need to start consistently doing the one or two things that are most important for your health *right now*.

We'll talk a lot about what those steps and tiny changes should be for you in the coming pages. They can be different for everyone, depending on where you are with your health and what you've done in the past. But for the vast majority of people, it comes down to just picking one or two of what we call the Four Core Actions—and sticking with just those until they become automated, effortless habits.

It's essential to relax, have treats, go on date night, brunch with friends, and have fun. We *need* these things in our lives. This is one of the most important elements of *balance* in the Alkaline Life.

This is the first of the two concepts of balance.

The other essential balance is the balance *within your body*.

Your body craves balance. There are myriad balances that need to be maintained throughout what I call your Five Master Systems: the immune, endocrine, digestive, detoxification, and pH buffering systems.* And it's your body's pH that is the foundation of everything.

We call it the Alkaline Life because the pH of your blood *must* be maintained at a slightly alkaline level. The optimal level is pH 7.365, and the body will do anything and everything to ensure that it does not fall far below this level.[9] If it does, you will die quite quickly. It is that important. When your body has to drop everything and anything to focus on returning your blood to a safe pH over and over, the stress and imbalance it causes everywhere else in the body is devastating.

As I've mentioned, practically every disease can be traced back to excess acidity and the stress caused by the body having to constantly buffer your blood pH. Cancer,[10] heart disease,[11] type 2 diabetes,[12] and strokes[13] all have excess acidity either directly or indirectly at the root of the problem.

But as we get into what the Alkaline Life looks like and what diet-induced acidity does to your body, I want you to *always* keep front of mind:

a. the *only* thing you need to do is nourish your body.

b. you *never* need to be perfect.

80/20 AND THE MINIMUM EFFECTIVE DOSE

You've probably heard of the 80/20 rule before, known as the *Pareto principle*. It's a rule that can apply to practically everything

---

* I discuss the Five Master Systems in depth in my first book, *The Alkaline Reset Cleanse*.

in life, yet I don't know anybody applying it directly to healthy living and nutrition.

The Pareto principle is the concept that in any given situation or pursuit, 80 percent (or more) of the output is always a result of 20 percent (or less) of the inputs. We see it everywhere in everyday life:

1. In the workplace, 80 percent of the work is done by 20 percent of the employees.

2. In a business, 80 percent of the revenue comes from 20 percent of the customers.

3. In a city, 80 percent of the traffic is on 20 percent of the roads.

4. In personal finance, 80 percent of expenses comes from 20 percent of spending categories.

5. In the home, 80 percent of the mess comes from 20 percent of the activities.

And when it comes to *your* Alkaline Life, you can reach 80 percent of your goal with just 20 percent of the activities.

And rather than 80/20, I actually prefer to call this the 20/80, because it leans more into the concept that by focusing on the 20 percent of actions that have the biggest impact for you and making them into habits, you truly can get 80 percent of the way to your goal.

80 Percent Is the First Goal

To be clear, I am not suggesting we'll get you to 80 percent of your health goals and then stop. The aim with my 20/80 approach is to get you to 80 percent of your health goals as quickly and easily as possible.

Think now about one of your biggest health goals, and picture what it would be like if you were already 80 percent of the way there. What would your energy be like? What would your outlook and mood be like? How much better would you feel, move, and sleep? How much positivity would be in your life, and how much hope for the future?

Our aim together is to get you to that place as quickly and easily as possible. Once you're 80 percent of the way there, your energy and vitality will be such that achieving the remaining 20 percent of your goal will be easy! You'll feel so good, and have so much momentum, that taking the next steps will be desirable and exciting.

As we get started, I want you to keep this top of mind. It may seem simple at first, but I know from experience, **just a small number of seemingly little habits, practiced consistently, can yield huge results. They are the little levers that lift big weights.**

Most people dramatically overestimate what they can achieve in a day or a week but vastly underestimate what they can do in 14 days. If you apply the principles in this book and build them as habits over a 14-day period, you'll see results beyond what you could possibly have imagined.

All you need to do is just pick your first 20/80 actions, and that's where I can help. I'll guide you through each of these powerful moves, step-by-step, and give you everything you need to make it real, make it happen, and make it stick for life.

Karona's Story

I had been on letrozole (a cancer medication) for 18 months and lost so much hair. I felt sick all the time. An oncologist conceded to allowing me to go off this medication, but on the condition that I start tamoxifen immediately, which started another nightmare. The tamoxifen left me extremely nauseated and weak, and with such pain in my bones I could barely stand.

My baby sister (10 years younger) had stomach cancer. She wasn't into any form of health protocol and used chemotherapy *and* radiation. She was dead within a year. This is when I discovered the alkaline way.

Things turned around so quickly. Within no time, I had two consecutive days without wanting or needing to spend my days over the toilet, being paralyzed with nausea, and now this is my normal.

My friends from Vancouver, British Columbia, saw me last week and told me that they "never saw [me] look so good." They knew right away that something pretty significant had happened to me. This is *not* temporary! This will be for the rest of my life.

I have not felt like this in years. I am now medication-free with the support of my wonderful general practitioner and thriving.

· CHAPTER 2 ·

Living in Balance:
The Science behind
the Alkaline Life

When it comes to our health, it's important to understand the basics of the science behind why we do what we do.

The importance of blood pH and our body's requirement to maintain its delicate balance has long been understood.

In the 19th century, trailblazing practitioners such as Franz Xaver Mayr (who was famed for introducing his *F. X. Mayr Kur*, a method of natural intestinal cleansing) introduced the concept of balancing acids by eating foods with an excess of alkali. But they were well ahead of the technology that could prove this, and therefore they were largely ignored.

While the first studies relating to blood pH and health (that I'm aware of) were published in 1917,[1] examining the relationship between alkalinity and diabetes, there were few definitive studies to truly examine the impact of dietary acids and the benefits of eating alkaline-forming foods until the 1960s, when the technology to study blood acid-base status emerged.

Over the next 40 to 50 years, research trickled in, slowly building momentum. As we learned more about the mechanisms by which the body neutralizes acidity, the studies turned to the relationship between calcium loss and bone health.

When I first started to learn about, and then coach, the alkaline way back in 2003, pioneering researchers such as Dr. Lynda Frassetto and Dr. Joseph Pizzorno were leading the charge, but they were still met with skepticism.

And the arguments against following an alkaline approach to health that were published in 1936[2] *are still being used today* by pop nutritionists, influencers, and sadly, those who have not kept up to date with current research in the medical field.[3]

In the 1936 paper, the author argued, "Faddists rampant in the realm of pseudo-science have seized upon the acid-base balance of the body as an apt subject for their sophistry . . . the acid-base balance is maintained in a definite state of equilibrium . . . the effects of food on this balance have been greatly exaggerated, for their influence . . . is practically nil."

This argument, which may have been justifiable almost a hundred years ago without the knowledge and tools we have now, is basically, "the body has its own pH-buffering mechanisms; diet won't change that." Inexplicably, critics of the alkaline approach are still saying this, despite the abundance of studies and data we have now proving that diet is essential to the acid-base balance in the body and relates to dozens of health conditions, as shown in studies in *The American Journal of Clinical Nutrition*,[4] the *Nutrition Journal*,[5] the *British Journal of Nutrition*,[6] *Nutrition & Metabolism*,[7] *Clinical Nutrition*,[8] and so many more (this book references over 200 of these studies, and we're just scratching the surface!).

Over the next couple of chapters, we are going to dig into the actual science, studies, and truth about the Alkaline Life, and how it relates to our practical steps, to put it into practice. I'll explain the scientific mechanisms and supporting research in a very user-friendly way, and everything is referenced in case you want to read some of the studies like I do. I'm an ex-academic who *loves* the studies and the data!

WHAT IT MEANS TO "LIVE ALKALINE"

Before we dig into the science, I want to explain what it means to "live alkaline" in the simplest way possible:

> To live alkaline, you should focus 80 percent or more of your diet on foods that are alkaline forming and keep the acid-forming part of your food and drink intake below 20 percent.

See? Simple!

Note that I say alkaline *forming* and acid *forming*. This is important.

Focus 80 percent of your diet on alkaline-forming foods such as vegetables, fruits, nuts, seeds, healthy fats, leafy greens, oily fish, herbs and spices, and proper hydration. Foods like salads, avocados, cucumbers, broccoli, celery, bell pepper, spinach, kale, blueberries, carrots, beets, oats, quinoa, lettuce—you get the picture.

The acid-forming foods to keep in your 20 percent bucket include sugar, gluten, processed foods, fast foods, trans fats, refined foods, and packaged food. These are things like chips, pizza, soda, artificial sweeteners, processed meats, cookies, cakes, sweets—again, you get the picture.

There are, of course, nuances and a little more to it than this, but this is what the alkaline approach is at a very high level. Don't worry, we'll get into all the details you need to know (and none that you don't), but I want to give you a simple set of guiding principles, a foundation, that you can always come back to if you ever get lost.

It is, of course, important to recognize that not everyone is the same, and I truly do believe that one *size fits one*. However, supporting your body to balance your pH is perhaps *the* most powerful thing you can do to prevent sickness and disease and allow your body to thrive with energy and vitality.

It's Not about Being *More* Alkaline

This might surprise you, but we are not trying to make your body *more* alkaline, and it is not about *changing* your pH. This is essential to remember.

Wait . . . what?

That's right. The Alkaline Life is not about changing your pH to make your body *more* alkaline. This is not our goal.

The goal of the Alkaline Life is to support your body to maintain the perfectly balanced pH levels throughout your organs, tissues, glands, cells, and extracellular fluids, with the most important being the slightly alkaline pH of the blood, at close to pH 7.365.

The foods we eat, the drinks we drink, the way we live—all have a direct and dramatic impact on the body's ability to maintain this pH.

If we eat a "standard modern diet"* (SMD) of processed foods, sugar, caffeine, unhealthy fats, dairy, gluten, and so on, we are constantly plunging our blood pH down, and it causes a huge stress to the body to upregulate it back to that pH of 7.365.

The body will do whatever it takes to keep your blood pH in a tight range around 7.365. Again, it will drop everything and do *anything* to keep the pH at this slightly alkaline level.

Why? Well, if your blood pH drops below this level, you die.[9]

It's as simple as that. You can't do anything about this. You can eat as acidic as you like; you can eat only acidic foods and drink only the most acidic drinks (diet soda, in case you're wondering), and your body will *always* regulate your pH back to a safe level.[10]

You might be thinking, *Hang on, the 1936 study mentioned earlier was right! If my body is going to do this balancing anyway, why do we need to eat alkaline? And why should I worry about it?*

It's a fair question, and it does seem intuitive, right? If your body keeps your blood alkaline anyway, why stress about it? In fact, this is perhaps the most common misunderstanding of the alkaline approach that critics have.

But while it's true to say that the body regulates your pH and you can't change it, *this is exactly the point.*

Our goal is to provide your body with a diet and lifestyle that doesn't overload it with acidity to deal with while also nourishing

---

* I know everybody calls it the "standard American diet," or SAD, but the rest of the world doesn't get off that easily! The diet in the U.K., Europe, Australia, and elsewhere is similar to the SAD.

it with the alkaline-forming nutrients it needs to thrive. We don't want to *change* your pH; we want to support the body to maintain it without the stress that diet-induced acidity causes.

WE WERE NOT DESIGNED FOR THE STANDARD MODERN DIET!

When your body is constantly bombarded with acidity and your blood pH is driven down, it causes a huge amount of stress to your health. Bringing your pH back from acidic to alkaline impacts every area of your body, from your hormones[11] to your digestion[12] and from your liver[13] to your kidneys.[14]

While we have evolved with a small acid-buffering capacity, this is no match for the SMD. This buffering capacity, which largely consists of increasing bicarbonate, proteins, and phosphate,[15] is able to manage only the tiny amount of acidity produced naturally by our daily bodily functions. It wasn't designed for a bacon-and-egg bagel, a large mocha, and OJ before we've left the house in the morning!

To take a quick step back and transport you in time to your middle-school science lessons (hello, Mr. Rose!), the pH scale runs from pH 1 to pH 14. pH 7 is neutral, and anything lower is acidic, while anything higher is alkaline.

As we dig deeper into the depths of our middle-school memories, we might remember too that the pH scale is logarithmic. In simple terms, this means that anything with a pH of 6 (white rice, for example) is 10 times more acidic than a substance with a pH of 7 (such as oats). A substance with a pH of 5 (fruit jam) is 100 times more acidic. A pH of 4 is 1,000 times more acidic than a pH of 7, and so on. Cola and coffee have a pH of 3. Yes, they are 10,000 times more acid forming than neutral foods and drinks with a pH of 7.

You can see just how quickly the pH buffering capacity can be exhausted by our modern diet. Again, we evolved to be able to buffer the acidity made by our metabolism, but now we're throwing down soda, cappuccinos, pizza, chips, and ice cream and expecting the body to cope.

It can't.

Once our initial buffering capacity has been exhausted (about halfway through the third mouthful of that breakfast we talked about), we start getting into trouble.

Our next line of defense is the lungs and kidneys, which become significantly stressed by having to perform this role day in and day out. The lungs boost blood pH by increasing respiration (your rate of breathing) to reduce excess carbon dioxide.

The kidneys then kick in with two mechanisms. The body reabsorbs more bicarbonate (HCO_3^-) from the urine and puts it back into the blood. Then, the liver produces more ammonia, which then reacts with acids to create ammonium. The kidneys have to excrete this, thus getting the acids out and increasing blood pH.[16]

This line of defense is just as quickly worn out, and the stress of raising pH causes significant imbalance to the kidneys, liver, and lungs.

Once these three lines of defense have been defeated, the body takes drastic measures—we're in big trouble now. Alkaline minerals, including calcium, magnesium, sodium, potassium, and zinc are taken from the bones, muscles, and more;[17] they are then released into the bloodstream.[18] This process is called *remineralization*.

This is catastrophic to the body. A powerful example is its negative impact on bone density. Dozens upon dozens of studies have demonstrated that excess dietary acidity is strongly correlated with osteoporosis risk. This makes total sense. If we keep consuming acid-forming foods, the body has to draw alkaline minerals from the bone tissue, and the bones become weaker.[19, 20, 21, 22, 23, 24, 25]

Another outcome of the overreliance on these buffering mechanisms is an increased risk of kidney stones. When the body pulls alkaline minerals into the blood, the increased calcium can form hard mineral deposits in the kidneys or urinary tract.[26, 27, 28, 29]

And we're only just getting started with the damage of diet-induced acidosis. If you're ready for the scary stuff, let's get into it.

Gina's Story

What brought me to the alkaline life to begin with was a very rough road since I turned 36. I'm a two-time cancer survivor, but the chemotherapy that I had to go through caused neuropathy in both of my legs and chemo brain. I have acid reflux gastroparesis and a lower immunity system now because of the chemo and many other things going on in my body.

Of course, it isn't always just one straight, easy road, but the challenges are more manageable now than what they were before.

Once I started, I lost 20 pounds (9 kg) in four weeks. And I kept it off! And it really hasn't been hard to do. My reflux has cleared, and I feel my immunity is strong now. I don't get sick anymore.

My thinking is clearer, and all of the brain fog has gone. I love the way it makes me feel. Getting all of those vegetables and nuts and everything else that's so good for my body gives me so much energy. It gives me life again, a zest to live. It also makes it so that I'm able to keep the weight off and be able to look in the mirror and see the me that I've loved for so many years.

It's a journey, and it's one I'm looking forward to now. My recommendation to everyone is to live the alkaline way, and I promise you, you will love it every step of the way.

· CHAPTER 3 ·

Diet-Induced Acidosis and the "Safe Zone"

You've just learned about the body's three lines of defense against the acidic standard modern diet. If you think that's already scary and eye-opening, brace yourself for what's about to come!

The damage of an acidic diet is most definitely not confined to just the stress caused by regulating pH back to where it needs to be. It's not just the stress to the liver, kidneys, and lungs and the borrowing of alkaline minerals from your bones and muscles that we discussed in Chapter 2. It's far more insidious than this.

Due to how stressful it is for your body to raise your blood pH all the way back to the ideal pH 7.365, your body can only raise it to a level that is "safe"—but this is far from optimal.

Your pH-buffering mechanisms will kick in, but your body won't get your pH all the way back to optimal—just to a "safe" level hovering a couple of points just below the optimal pH of 7.365. In the scientific literature, this is called *diet-induced metabolic acidosis.*[1, 2, 3]

Remember, if your blood pH drops just a little below pH 7.365, you will die. So your body gets to a place where you are safe from immediately dying, but you don't want to live there. In a state of diet-induced acidosis (DIA), sickness and disease proliferate.

Increased risk of cancer,[4, 5] atherosclerosis,[6] autoimmune disease,[7] stroke,[8] osteoporosis,[9] chronic kidney disease,[10] nonalcoholic fatty liver disease (NAFLD),[11] and immune disorders[12] are all rooted in diet-induced acidosis, aka the "safe" zone.

And yet, this is where most people are living—all day, every day. From the moment they wake, their body is in a state of DIA from processing acidity from the night before. Then their acid-forming breakfast of bread, caffeine, preserves, processed meats, fruit juice, and sugar drives blood pH lower. And from here it is a vicious cycle throughout the day. There is no respite. The body is in a state of constant stress.

When we're living in DIA, the impact on our digestive system, cardiovascular system, immune system, detoxification system, and endocrine system is huge.

Again, it's not just the excess acidity that is problematic (which is the primary cause of gout, reflux, and gut dysbiosis), or the secondary problems this causes (such as inflammation and oxidative stress), but there are layers and layers of problems that all begin with diet-induced acidosis at the root.

In a case-control study published in 2021,[13] researchers found a direct link between dietary acid load and lung cancer risk in men. Looking at 843 lung cancer cases, they found that diet-induced acidosis created a cascade of issues, including a disruption of enzyme function, loss of insulin sensitivity, cellular adaptations, tissue damage, blocking of immune functions, inflammation, and inflammation-induced oxidative stress, which in turn triggered DNA damage and cell mutation. These factors, both independently and combined, dramatically increased cancer risk.

And in a cross-sectional study[14] looking at 11,601 subjects, researchers found that those who had the highest acid-forming diet had a far greater risk of cardiovascular disease (CVD), independent of the normal risk factors such as weight. Again, the causes were multilayered. The study showed the mechanism for this increased CVD risk was due to diet-induced acidosis causing rapid insulin resistance, potassium deficiency (remember, buffering blood pH requires potassium to be pulled from the body) leading to blood vessel toxicity and chronically elevated cortisol levels, and the loss of renal function and an increased risk of arrhythmogenesis.

And a study[15] looking at the link between diet-induced acidosis and nonalcoholic fatty liver disease, including 5,967 participants, found that the impacts of DIA that led to increased risk included endocrine imbalance (particularly of the hypothalamic-pituitary-adrenal axis), increases in intestinal permeability and visceral fat cell formation, an excess of sulfur-containing amino acids damaging the liver directly, growth hormone imbalance, and, again, causing insulin sensitivity.

This is just three studies looking at three primary outcomes. You can see that diet-induced acidosis is scary. Just in these studies, we've seen it cause tissue damage, insulin insensitivity, DNA damage, hormone imbalance, cell mutation, mineral deficiency, adrenal stress, an increase of fat cells, and liver damage.

From these three studies (and there are thousands more like them), you can see that each of the Five Master Systems of the digestive, endocrine, immune, detoxification, and pH buffering systems are seriously impacted.

Depending on the goals or challenges you have right now, reaching your ultimate goal could take weeks, or it could take months—but it takes only days to start seeing impactful results. I'm here to support you and to make the journey as easy, enjoyable, and fun as possible.

The Spiral of Diet-Induced Acidity

The direct impact of diet-induced acidity is not the only concern. For each imbalance, there is a flow-on effect. When imbalance occurs in one area, it quickly creates a new set of imbalances and challenges in other areas. It is all intricately linked.

A good example of this is DIA's impact on the regulation of cortisol. When we live in that (not-so-) safe zone of diet-induced acidosis, our adrenals pump out excess cortisol.[16] This causes incredible stress to the adrenal glands. If we exert it on the adrenals 24/7, the result is not pretty. Impaired adrenal function can quickly lead to increased risk of obesity,[17] type 2 diabetes,[18] depression,[19] chronic kidney disease,[20] and more.

Chronic excess cortisol is driven largely by diet-induced acidosis, but here's the kicker: excess cortisol in the body also causes lower blood pH.[21]

It's a vicious cycle.

But worse, adrenal fatigue also leads to a cascade of other imbalances, such as of the pituitary gland, of the hypothalamus, and in the production of thyroid hormones. It promotes a slowed metabolism and impaired liver function. Each of these conditions then has its own flow-on effect to other areas of your health, which then need to be healed.

We must stop all of this at its root: diet-induced acidity.

INTRODUCING THE TRIPLE-A

In the studies I've shared, you will have seen three outcomes come up over and over: acidity, inflammation, and oxidative stress.

These three issues are at the root of every health challenge and disease. They are interlinked, and we need to address them all.

In recent times, there's been a lot more focus on the impact of chronic inflammation in the body. Conditions such as lupus, arthritis, inflammatory bowel disease (IBS), leaky gut, fibromyalgia, and psoriasis are all rooted in inflammation, and they have

DIA sitting behind them. And even more serious conditions such as cancer, type 2 diabetes, Alzheimer's disease, and kidney disease are all commonly associated with the presence of chronic inflammation too.

Inflammation is an entirely preventable disease through diet and lifestyle choices—but an acid-forming diet is like throwing gasoline on the fire.

Aging is effectively oxidative stress, which occurs when there's an imbalance between the production of molecules called *free radicals* and our body's ability to counteract their harmful effects. When we're in a state of DIA, oxidative stress increases radically,[22] damaging cells, proteins, and DNA in our body, which can contribute to aging and a variety of diseases such as heart disease, cancer, arthritis, stroke, respiratory diseases, immune deficiency, and neurodegenerative diseases like Alzheimer's.

Some describe oxidation as the "rusting" of the body, and just like rust corrodes metal when exposed to oxygen, our cells can be "corroded" when overexposed to those free radicals. Our body creates them naturally, but with DIA, they easily get out of balance.

But the solution to preventing DIA, inflammation, and oxidative stress is simple. It's what I call "the Triple-A."

And when we apply the Triple-A, things start to get good really quickly. Let's get into it.

· CHAPTER 4 ·

The Triple-A Foods to *Thrive*

The Alkaline Life is *alkaline, antioxidant rich, and powerfully anti-inflammatory*: the Triple-A. This is the perfect antidote to the acidity, oxidative stress, and inflammation that sits behind every sickness and disease. When we flood the body with alkaline, antioxidant-rich, anti-inflammatory foods—the "Triple-A" foods—we can rapidly undo the damage caused by the standard modern diet and rebalance, rebuild, and repair our health.

So, let's get started with the most important foods to focus on to get out of diet-induced acidosis and into optimal health.

WHAT WE EAT AND WHAT WE AVOID IN THE ALKALINE LIFE

It will be no surprise to hear that we'll be focusing our diet on a lot of alkaline-*forming* foods and reducing our intake (not completely) of acid-*forming* foods.

And if I were to give you a list of a hundred foods and say that alkaline-forming foods are "healthy" and acid-forming foods are generally "unhealthy," you'd probably be able to have a good stab at categorizing them into acidic or alkaline. But there's more detail and nuance to it than this. Did you notice that I didn't simply call the foods acidic and alkaline? As I mentioned earlier, and it is worth reiterating, the word *forming* is very important.

Why Are Lemons on the Alkaline List?

When you get to my acid and alkaline food charts, you'll see some seemingly odd and counterintuitive listings. And if you spend any time online looking at the food charts dotted around the Internet, you'll see a fair amount of variation. Some say a food is alkaline and to eat as much of it as you like, and others say it's acidic. So what's going on here? Isn't a food acidic or alkaline, and that's that?

Not quite.

When people first join the Alkaline Life Club, a question they ask me a lot is, "Lemons are acidic, so why are you saying they're alkaline?" The explanation is simple and covers many of the seemingly counterintuitive foods on the alkaline list, including lemons, limes, tomatoes, and several other fruits and vegetables: we're not concerned by whether a food is alkaline or acidic in nature, on the tree or plant. *We're only concerned with the impact it has on the body once digested.*

This is why it's important to understand the distinction of alkaline- or acid-*forming.*

Using lemons as an example, the citric acid in lemon juice means that in nature, outside of the body, it's acidic. Now, not only is citric acid a "weak" acid—meaning it is quickly metabolized and broken down into its basic components without any real impact on our pH—but the body breaks down and metabolizes lemon, releasing its strong alkaline mineral content including calcium, potassium, and magnesium. The net result is a mildly alkaline-forming effect on the body.

Another good example is bananas, which are often misrepresented as alkaline in food charts. While bananas do have reasonable levels of the alkaline mineral potassium, they are incredibly high in fructose, which, once metabolized by the liver, creates a ton of uric acid, leaving an acidic effect on the body that far outweighs the potassium content.

This concept of acid- or alkaline-forming explains most of the differences between the information I'm giving you and what's in the other charts of acid and alkaline foods you'll see out there.

The contradictions between food charts is one of the biggest sources of confusion and frustration for many of my new students when they join the Alkaline Life Club. They see on one food chart that oranges are alkaline, but on another, they're acidic. On one chart, mushrooms are alkaline and on another, acidic.

Most of this is due to a chart using *only* the potential renal acid load (PRAL)[1] methodology of assessing the alkaline- or acid-forming potential of a food, whereas you really need to also use the net endogenous acid production[2] (NEAP) method too, and then overlay the factors that neither of these methods can pick up.

The main shortfalls of these methods are that they don't pick up the fact that the following components of foods are very acid forming:

- **Fungi.** All fungi are acid forming, meaning that mushrooms, even medicinal ones, don't support your pH balance. Medicinal mushrooms such as chaga, lion's mane, and so on can be used short term to assist with specific health goals, but they are not foods you should be consuming day-to-day.

- **Algae.** All algae are acid forming, so spirulina and chlorella are not the best sources of greens.

- **Yeasts.** The acid-forming nature of yeasts eliminates breads and gluten-containing grains from an alkaline diet.

- **Fructose.** This is a slightly more complex one, but concentrated fructose, such as from juiced fruit, dried fruit, and syrups, is highly acid forming.

- **Mycotoxins.** Present in certain foods, like peanuts, mycotoxins feed bacteria in the blood and drive blood pH down.

Most contradictions and inconsistencies with regard to food charts involve these components. High-sugar fruits and fruit juices, syrups and honey, mushrooms, spirulina, chlorella, nutritional yeast, fermented foods, and peanuts are the most common foods to be incorrectly categorized as alkaline forming.

There is a fairly comprehensive acid-and-alkaline-forming food chart in Part IV of this book, but for a clear, definitive list of over 400 acid and alkaline foods ranked and categorized from strongly acid forming through neutral and all the way to strongly alkaline forming, I recommend you head to www .thealkalinelifebook.com and download my charts for free. Throughout this book, whenever I refer to foods as acid and alkaline, the terms *acid forming* and *alkaline forming* apply.

My alkaline food charts have been developed over almost two decades. My process:

1. Uses PRAL as a starting point
2. Overlays NEAP to iron out inconsistencies
3. Adjusts for sugar content and the other components listed above
4. Factors in the food's natural-state pH
5. Accounts for the food's mineral content
6. Considers the effect the food has instantaneously on the blood once consumed (as per blood microscopy)

I believe this makes my charts the most reliable and accurate available.

However, the most important thing here, again, is to not get too bogged down in the minutiae or worry about being perfect. You don't need to eat only alkaline foods forever. You can have some acid-forming foods, and if you make the odd mistake, it's not a big deal.

Approach the Alkaline Life with relaxed confidence, knowing that I am going to give you the step-by-step guidance to make it simple and easy.

Get 400+ Foods Ranked from Acid to Alkaline

In my definitive Acid/Alkaline Food Chart (page 282), I've ranked over 400 foods and drinks from strongly acid forming through to neutral and on to strongly alkaline forming.

It's the ultimate guide and also comes with a one-page, at-a-glance, printer-friendly acid/alkaline chart to stick on your fridge! Download it at www.thealkalinelifebook.com.

THE GOOD STUFF: HIGH ALKALINE FOODS AND NUTRIENTS TO ENERGIZE AND THRIVE

As we've discussed, living the Alkaline Life is simple: focus on consuming *mostly* alkaline-forming foods and reduce your intake of acid-forming foods. Some like to think of this as 80/20 (80 percent alkaline-forming foods and 20 percent acid forming), and if that helps you, then you can do this too. I find it easier to simply use intuition and ballpark estimates that most of my food intake is alkaline forming. Don't underestimate your intuition.

As we get into the most alkaline foods, you'll quickly see that the balance *is* largely intuitive. If I gave a hundred people a big list of random foods and asked them to group them into acid forming or alkaline forming, 95 percent of them would get it 95 percent right. The Alkaline Life makes total sense and uses the power of nature to heal and rebalance our body.

Of course, some foods are more nutrient dense than others, so I've focused on these to give you the maximum bang for your buck and speed the healing process as much as possible.

Don't worry about recipes just yet—you have lots of delicious meals in Part IV to try. I have been creating alkaline recipes for close to 20 years, and the ones in this book will knock your socks off, soon to become firm family favorites. And as you go through my food list, don't worry if I mention certain ones you don't currently love or haven't eaten before. Instead, I want you to remember that there are so many delicious alkaline foods and easy substitutes for any food you can't currently tolerate or don't like. Again, there's a *lot* of flexibility in my Alkaline Life Plan.

These are the foods I want you to focus on:

- Leafy greens
- Antioxidant-rich vegetables
- Raw nuts and seeds
- Healthy fats and oils
- Anti-inflammatory foods
- Alkaline protein
- Low-sugar fruits

Let's look at them in a bit of depth now.

LEAFY GREENS

The standard government guidelines in most countries fall something along the lines of "five servings per day of fruits and vegetables." Sadly, not only do most people get nowhere near this,[3,4] even including fruit, but this recommendation is nowhere near what you need to thrive. Rather than five a day, I would *love it* if they changed the recommendation to five a day or more of *leafy greens!*

Leafy greens are *the* most nutrient-dense foods on earth. In my first book, *The Alkaline Reset Cleanse*, I referenced a study called "Defining Powerhouse Fruits and Vegetables,"[5] which examined the micronutrient content of lots of different foods and ranked the top 41 (not sure why 41!) most nutrient-dense foods. The top 15 are *all* leafy greens.

When we talk about how 20 percent of your actions can give you 80 percent of the results you desire, adding 5 to 7 servings of leafy greens per day is perhaps the most powerful and efficient thing you can do. Spinach, kale, watercress, lettuce, chard, silver beet, and beet greens are all so powerfully nutritious, with an incredible range of vitamins, minerals, antioxidants, protein, healthy fats, and fiber.

Leafy greens to focus on: kale, spinach, watercress, cabbage, lettuce, beet greens, chard, arugula, collards, and bok choy.

In Part III I give you all the steps to build the habit of getting 5 to 7 servings of leafy greens a day and put it on autopilot. For now, I want you to know that these foods are essential and incredibly beneficial.

The more unique nutrients contained in leafy greens include the following.

Chlorophyll

Chlorophyll is a green pigment present in all green vegetables, especially leafy greens. While chlorophyll is best known for its role in photosynthesis, it is *amazing* for our health. It ticks all three boxes of being highly alkaline-forming, antioxidant rich, and powerfully anti-inflammatory.

Chlorophyll is a powerful natural detoxifier that has been shown to bind to and remove toxins, such as heavy metals and environmental pollutants, from the body.[6]

It is healing for the digestive system,[7] has anti-aging benefits, is anti-inflammatory,[8] neuroprotective,[9] and is great for the skin.[10] Plus, research has shown that it can reduce the risk of several cancers.[11]

Sulforaphane

Sulforaphane, a compound found in cruciferous vegetables such as broccoli and kale, has been shown to have a variety of health benefits, including the ability to protect and support the immune system.[12]

One way that sulforaphane does this is by activating the NRF2 pathway.[13] NRF2 triggers the production of antioxidant enzymes and other molecules that protect the body's cells from damage caused by free radicals.

Studies have shown that sulforaphane can improve the function of immune cells such as T cells and natural killer cells, and it may also help reduce inflammation in the body.[14]

In addition to its effects on the immune system, sulforaphane has been studied for its potential benefits for a variety of health conditions, including cancer, heart disease, and neurodegenerative diseases like Alzheimer's and Parkinson's.[15]

Unique Antioxidant Mix

We're going to look a little deeper at antioxidant-rich foods in a minute, but I want to touch on the unique and powerful antioxidants that can be found only in dark, leafy greens. Their combination of carotenoids and flavonoids makes them an incredibly powerful source of antioxidants, which have strong anti-inflammatory properties.

Carotenoids are a group of antioxidants that give fruits and vegetables their vibrant colors. Dark, leafy greens like spinach and kale are particularly rich in carotenoids like lutein, zeaxanthin, and beta-carotene.

Flavonoids are a diverse group of antioxidants that have been shown to have anti-inflammatory, anticancer, and heart-protective properties.[16]

Dark, leafy greens like kale and Swiss chard are particularly high in flavonoids like quercetin and kaempferol, which have been linked to a reduced risk of heart disease. One of quercetin's unique benefits is its ability to reduce and remove allergy symptoms, and kaempferol is incredibly neuroprotective.[17]

They are also rich in glucosinolates, which are essential precursors to sulforaphane production and react with myrosinase, a type of enzyme, to produce a powerfully strong anticancer effect.[18]

Leafy greens are a source of some of the most potent anticancer antioxidants, known as *betalains*. Betalains are found only in leafy greens, beets, dragonfruit, and prickly pear, so eating greens is a great way to make sure you're getting enough of this important nutrient.[19]

I also want to give a quick mention of the omega-3 content of leafy greens. While they are not as high in healthy fats compared to fish or nuts, they are a valuable additional source. On average, 5 servings of leafy greens would provide you with around 500 to 700 milligrams of omega-3. When you consider that the average recommended dietary intake (RDI) for omega-3 is 1.1 grams for women and 1.6 grams for men, leafy greens would be a great boost!

The Truth about Oxalate, Nightshades, and "Antinutrients"

I want to very quickly dispel any myths and lies about oxalate, nightshades, and so-called antinutrients.

Let's tackle them one by one.

Oxalate: I admit, on paper, it would be easy to believe that excess oxalate can cause kidney stones. However, this is misleading and only a tiny piece of the picture. First, alkaline-forming greens containing oxalate, including spinach and kale, have actually been proven to *decrease* kidney stone risk[20] due to their nutrient content. These greens are high in calcium (which binds to oxalate in the gut and prevents it being absorbed), magnesium, and potassium. And yes, you've probably noted that these are all high-alkaline minerals.

A study published in the *Journal of the American Society of Nephrology*, using a data set of over 240,000 people tracked over 44 combined years, found that direct dietary oxalate accounts only for around 10 percent of the oxalate found in the urine of stone developers.[21] The oxalate is being formed in the body not from the foods we eat but because of *acid imbalances*.

Here are two quick examples: foods that contain phosphoric acid, such as processed meats, processed dairy, soda, baked goods, and many alcohols reduce the level of citrate in the urine, increasing stone risk.[22] And, high-sugar foods increase insulin levels, and insulin levels increase oxalate levels and risk of stone formation.[23]

Plus, studies show that antibiotic use destroys many beneficial gut bacteria, including *O. formigenes*, an oxalate-degrading bacteria, and other bacteria that increase oxalate excretion.[24]

As you can see, the cause of kidney stones is far more complex than simply the amount of oxalate you consume. Dietary oxalate is only ever going to have a very negligible impact, if any.

Nightshades: I think a lot of the fear here has come from the fact that this group of fruits and vegetables are called "deadly" nightshades! Scary name! However, similar to oxalates, the impact from dietary nightshade consumption is negligible at best. The "dotted line" theory here is that nightshades contain alkaloids called *solanine* and *chaconine*, which are there to act as a defense mechanism against insects and other predators, and some say these compounds overly trigger the immune system, contributing to autoimmune conditions.

However, the levels of these alkaloids in nightshade foods are absolutely tiny. Old white potatoes that have been left to sprout are the only food that would have even a slight risk, and you would have to eat a *lot* of old white potatoes to move the needle.

Data shows that the anti-inflammatory properties of nightshade vegetables, such as bell pepper, actually *reduce* the risk and severity of autoimmune conditions.[25]

Antinutrients: again, what's in a name? *Antinutrients.* Sounds aggressive and scary! *Antinutrients* is a term first coined in the 1960s and was related to several groups of substances, including drugs and environmental toxins, that could inhibit nutrient absorption and were used in all manner of applications such as agriculture and medicine. It was more commonly used as the name for a substance such as refined sugar or alcohol, that has little nutritive value and depletes the body of more nutrients than it provides when metabolized. It has been picked up in more recent times and used as a shock tactic for clicks and attention, with the exaggeration that eating certain foods will "leach minerals from your body."

The reality is while there is some truth to the fact that certain foods, such as spinach, oats, legumes, and nuts, *can* block the absorption of a small number of minerals, including calcium, zinc, and iron, when you dig a little deeper you quickly see that there are several important facts to consider. One is that the impact is tiny. You would have to eat absurd amounts of these foods to get any noticeable impact on your nutrient levels.[26]

The second fact is that the impact of these foods on nutrient absorption occurs only *during that particular meal*. It is a tiny impact, if any, that occurs in a very tiny window of your day.[27]

If you consume an even moderately varied diet, you'll be nowhere near deficient in zinc, iron, magnesium, or any other nutrients.

A so-called antinutrient food such as spinach, which is incredibly rich in magnesium, does not lead to a net loss of magnesium. Sure, maybe some of the magnesium in that meal will not be as bioavailable, but you'll still get a ton of magnesium from it. Whereas when you consume sugar, the kidneys are forced to excrete a huge amount of magnesium from the body in your urine. With sugar, there's an actual magnesium loss.[28]

A review published in 2020 in the gold-standard journal *Nutrients*[29] examined over 270 studies on antinutrients and could not find any conclusive evidence of a deleterious effect on human health. In fact, the study concluded, "what has been referred to as 'anti-nutrients,' may, in fact, be therapeutic agents for various conditions."

And this is the real risk. By eliminating these foods for their almost nonexistent risk, you'll be missing out on absolutely critical nutrients and a lot of delicious foods!

If you want a deeper dive into the data and studies, go to www .thealkalinelifebook.com/oxalate.

ANTIOXIDANT-RICH VEGGIES

As part of the Triple-A, antioxidants help protect the body from damage caused by oxidative stress. As we already discussed, oxidative stress contributes to aging and increases the risk of a wide range of chronic diseases, such as cancer, heart disease, and Alzheimer's disease.

Antioxidants work by neutralizing free radicals and preventing them from causing damage to cells and tissues. They do this by donating an electron to the free radical, which stabilizes the molecule and prevents it from reacting with other molecules in the body.

> Antioxidant-rich foods to focus on: bell pepper, tomato, carrot, onion, garlic, leafy greens, turmeric, ginger, blueberries, avocado, broccoli, cauliflower, and sweet potato.

Antioxidants can be incredibly powerful. Most people will think of examples such as vitamin E and vitamin C, but there are dozens of powerful compounds that support our health:

- **Lycopene**—a carotenoid antioxidant found in red and pink fruits and vegetables, such as tomatoes and pink grapefruit, that helps protect against cancer[30] and heart disease[31] and helps reduce inflammation in the body
- **Quercetin**—a flavonoid antioxidant found in onions and kale that helps reduce inflammation and allergy symptoms and supports healthy immune function[32]
- **Coenzyme Q10**—a natural antioxidant found in every cell in the body that helps protect against free-radical damage, supports heart health, and helps reduce inflammation[33]
- **Alpha-lipoic acid**—an antioxidant that can help regenerate other antioxidants in the body, supports healthy glucose metabolism, and has anti-inflammatory effects[34]

- **Carotenoids**—a group of antioxidants that include beta-carotene, lutein, and zeaxanthin; it supports eye health and skin health, helps protect against cancer and heart disease, and helps reduce inflammation in the body.[35]

A special mention should go to glutathione too. Known as the "master antioxidant," glutathione is incredibly unique, important, and frankly amazing. It is a tripeptide composed of three amino acids—cysteine, glutamic acid, and glycine—and it not only plays a central role in protecting the body against free-radical damage but can also *regenerate* other antioxidants, such as vitamins C and E, that have been used up in the process of neutralizing free radicals. It can also help remove toxins and heavy metals,[36] reduce inflammation,[37] support liver function,[38] and reduce the risk of chronic disease and neurological disorders.[39]

Glutathione is an antioxidant that the body itself manufactures, and our ability to create it drops dramatically as we age. But the good news is, several alkaline-forming foods contain the building-block nutrients that our body can use to support glutathione production. The most important is avocado, which contains both glutamic acid and cystine. Other foods that support glutathione production include garlic, spinach, walnuts, and broccoli. All delicious, and all alkaline.

Broccoli Sprouts: The Sulforaphane Powerhouse

Sulforaphane has come up a few times already, and if there's one "niche" thing I would love you to try, it's growing your own sprouts—ideally, broccoli sprouts. When I began experimenting with the alkaline way, my friends and family officially started questioning me when I started sprouting. I got a bit obsessed, with dozens of jars on windowsills all over the house, each sprouting a different seed or blend.

I've chilled out a bit now and focus a lot of my sprouting specifically on broccoli sprouts. Broccoli sprouts contain 10 to 100 times the sulforaphane levels of the mature plant.[40] They also contain high levels of the precursor compound glucoraphanin and the enzyme myrosinase, which means that they provide a concentrated dose of sulforaphane that the body easily absorbs.

If you can add broccoli sprouts to your juices, smoothies, salads, stir-fries, soups, and sauces, you'll find a way to get a huge hit of sulforaphane daily.

I know it would be easy to dismiss this and put it in the "too hard" basket, but honestly, there are few compounds as powerful as sulforaphane. And broccoli sprouts give you a huge hit every day. Give it a try! This is a brilliant example of 20/80 in action.

RAW NUTS AND SEEDS

Nuts and seeds are both an excellent source of nutrients and a brilliant way to add delicious flavors, textures, and variety to recipes.

Nuts

Raw nuts are a great source of protein, healthy fats, antioxidants, and fiber. They make an incredible quick, on-the-go snack and can be used in so many alkaline desserts and to make delicious nut milks too.

Consuming raw, organic nuts can help reduce the risk of heart disease, lower blood pressure, and maintain a healthy cholesterol balance.

Some of my favorite nuts and their benefits include:

- **Brazil nuts**—one of the best sources of selenium—which boosts the immune system,[41] supports thyroid function,[42] reduces cancer risk,[43] and promotes brain health[44]
- **Walnuts**—a dense source of omega-3, vitamin E, B vitamins, magnesium, phosphorus, and copper. Fantastic for brain health,[45] heart health,[46] and support weight loss.[47]

- **Almonds**—an excellent source of fats, protein, fiber, vitamin E, magnesium, and potassium
- **Pecans**—an excellent source of healthy fats, fiber, and minerals such as zinc, manganese, and copper
- **Cashews**—which are rich in healthy fats, protein, fiber, and minerals such as magnesium, copper, and iron

Practically all nuts are alkaline forming and nutrient dense. The only nuts you need to avoid are peanuts. And while peanuts are officially legumes, most people consider them nuts, and use them like a nut, so they are included here! Peanuts should be avoided because they're incredibly vulnerable to mold during the growing, harvesting, and storage phase. One mold, a carcinogen called *aflatoxin*, is very concerning. Aflatoxin consumption is strongly linked to cancer and can cause liver toxicity. It is especially dangerous for pregnant women.[48]

Acid-forming molds have no place in an alkaline diet, and mold is one of the acid-forming things we're trying to avoid!

> Nuts to focus on: Brazil nuts, walnuts, pecans, almonds (be careful of volume, as these are high in omega-6), pistachios, hazelnuts, cashews, and macadamia nuts.

Seeds

Raw seeds are a fantastic inclusion to the alkaline diet, both nutritionally and for their beautiful flavors and textures! I include pumpkin, sunflower, sesame, flax, and chia seeds in my recipes day in and day out. They are so easy to add to smoothies and breakfasts, to make crackers with, and to add to soups and curries. When you get into the recipes in Part IV, you'll be pleasantly surprised at how often seeds are included when you least expect it.

- **Pumpkin seeds**—a great source of antioxidants, magnesium, zinc, and fatty acids. Interestingly, they also contain tryptophan, which is known for improving sleep quality.[49]

- **Sunflower seeds**—packed with healthy fats, protein, fiber, minerals, and vitamins. They contain high levels of vitamin E, a powerful antioxidant, and the alkaline minerals magnesium and selenium.

- **Sesame seeds**—a great source of lignans, which are strongly anticancer;[50] they can also help lower cholesterol[51] and blood pressure[52]

- **Flaxseeds**—well known for their high omega-3 fatty acid content, specifically alpha-linolenic acid (ALA), plus dietary fiber and lignans too. This combination of ALA, fiber, and lignans is why flax is lauded as such a powerful anticancer food.[53]

- **Chia seeds**—very high in fiber, protein, omega-3 fatty acids, and various micronutrients. The volume of protein with omega-3 makes them very useful on the Alkaline Life. Their gel-like texture once soaked also makes them incredibly versatile and useful for baking and making alkaline desserts!

- **Hemp seeds**—an excellent source of plant-based protein, providing all nine essential amino acids. They're also rich in omega-3 and omega-6 fatty acids in a well-balanced ratio. Additionally, they contain a good amount of fiber, vitamin E, and minerals.

Seeds to focus on: chia, pumpkin, sunflower, flax, hemp, and sesame.

HEALTHY FATS AND OILS

Fats and oils are critical to your health. They've been demonized and avoided in the modern diet for too long, and we need to embrace them and completely forget the notion that healthy fats are anything other than amazing for you.

Healthy fats and oils do not clog arteries, cause weight gain, or do any of the other things they've been wrongly accused of. The data is clear: healthy fats such as omega-3 and plant-based saturated fats from such sources as coconut *support heart health and weight loss!*

The messaging that demonized fats can be traced back to the now thoroughly debunked Seven Countries Study[54] by Ancel Keys that was commissioned to find the connection between diet and the increasing incidence of heart disease in the United States. Based on Keys's claims, the recommendations to cut fat from the diet were adopted by many countries, and it soon became a "known fact" that eating fat would cause heart disease and weight gain.

However, Keys's study was incredibly flawed, and countless studies both prior to and since Keys's paper have cleared healthy fats from the blame for the rise in heart disease, obesity, type 2 diabetes, cancer, and other degenerative diseases and placed it firmly at the door of sugar.

I know this is a challenging concept for some people to truly get behind. A lot of folks, when they first join the Alkaline Life Club, *believe* me when I tell them that fat does not make us gain weight and supports our cardiovascular health, but they just cannot bring themselves to eat it.

So, if you're in this position, I'll share just three studies to help.

In our first study, Dr. Rajiv Chowdhury and his team looked at 72 of the best studies on fat and heart disease (more than 600,000 people from 18 countries) and concluded there was no link between total fat or saturated fat and heart disease. They also found that trans fats increased, and omega-3 decreased, heart disease risk.[55]

The study also showed that two types of saturated fat linked to an increased risk of heart disease—palmitic and stearic acid—are *not* the saturated fats we eat. These two saturated fats can be made *only* in one, single way—as a toxic by-product of sugar being processed by the liver!

Study two, published in *The American Journal of Clinical Nutrition*, is another review, this time of 21 studies done with almost 350,000 people over a span of 23 years. It also showed saturated fat was not associated with increased risk of heart disease, heart attacks, stroke, or death.[56]

Study three, from the journal *Open Heart*, looked at all the randomized trials conducted up until the dietary guidelines denouncing fat were published by the United States government based on the Seven Countries Study, and *none* of the randomized trials showed that if you lowered fat, saturated fat, or dietary cholesterol, there was a reduction in heart disease.[57]

We could keep going with these for hours, but you get the picture. We have huge studies, massive data, and lack of evidence that healthy fats, including saturated fat, are a health risk.

We actually *need* healthy fats.

We'll delve into the specifics of unhealthy fats in the next chapter, but I want to stress the distinction between "good" and "bad" fats. Frankly, I wish we could label "bad" fats differently. They're so unlike "good" fats in their effects on our health that they could almost be considered an entirely separate category of substances.

Good fats and oils like olive oil, flax oil, chia seed oil, and the fats in foods such as nuts, seeds, avocado, fish, leafy greens, and so on are so incredibly beneficial. Bad fats, including seed oils such as sunflower and canola, are horribly toxic, as are margarine, trans fats, and hydrogenated fat. These are acid forming and cause imbalance and toxicity in the body.

Omega-3s to focus on: oily fish (salmon, tuna, mackerel, etc.), chia seeds, walnuts, hemp seeds, spinach, kale, brussels sprouts, and other leafy greens.

Fat Doesn't Make You Fat

Because the stuff stuck to your body is called "fat" and the stuff in our food is called "fat," we've been led to believe that eating fat makes us gain weight.

But this is absolutely, categorically not true. When you eat fat, it doesn't simply get stuck to your body. But because there's a multibillion-dollar *low-fat* industry constantly sending us messages that we need to eat less fat to lose weight, we believe it. We hear it over and over and over, and so it somehow becomes true, even though there's no actual data to support it.

Ironically, you're being fed this message while low-fat products are *filled* with sugar, preservatives, and chemicals, which actually contribute to making you gain weight and keeping it there.

This is important: weight gain is not caused by healthy fat consumption. It isn't caused by you eating omega-3 fatty acids, or even saturated fat. These fats help you to *lose* weight.

We'll dive into this more in Part III. However, I want you to fully understand that **weight gain is caused by imbalances in the body**—imbalances in thyroid and adrenal function, insulin management, inflammation, liver stress, digestive disorders, and so much more. In short, weight gain is one of many symptoms of living in the "safe" zone of diet-induced acidosis.

Weight Gain Comes from Imbalance

When we consume sugar (in particular, fructose), the liver becomes incredibly taxed. When the liver processes the fructose, there are several by-products. First, the liver creates a ton of uric acid. Chronically elevated uric acid levels then disrupt the body's ability to regulate blood sugar and insulin levels, leading to increased fat storage. The processing of fructose also creates a huge volume of inflammation, which encourages the body to create more visceral fat cells. The increased levels of pro-inflammatory cytokines, such as interleukin-6 (IL-6) and tumor necrosis factor alpha (TNF-α), encourage both the creation and storage of visceral fat around vital organs. These fat cells then become little inflamma-tion factories too, and a vicious cycle starts.

The inflammation from fructose metabolism also interferes with the normal function of adipose tissue, leading to changes in the expression of genes involved in fat metabolism and storage.

In short, with just one acid-forming food, you have six differ-ent ways that your body gains and clings to fat.

The bottom line is that fat does not make you gain weight. Acidic, toxic, inflammatory foods do. Alkaline, anti-inflammatory, antioxidant-rich foods do not. They will get you to your dream body weight, and this includes healthy fats!

A Bit about Cholesterol

The other big mental block people often have when it comes to eating healthy fats is about cholesterol. Again, we've been misled and told that cholesterol is bad and that eating fatty, cholesterol-rich foods will raise your cholesterol and increase your risk of cardiovascular disease. This is also simply not true, and all of the evidence is there to prove this.[58, 59, 60, 61]

The fact is, our body absolutely *needs* the vital substance of cholesterol to function properly. It's an essential component of cell membranes, and it's used to make hormones, vitamin D, and bile acids that help us digest fats. Our bodies can make all the choles-terol we need, and contrary to popular belief, the cholesterol we eat does not have a significant impact on our blood cholesterol lev-els. This is because our bodies regulate the amount of cholesterol in our bloodstream very tightly. When we eat cholesterol-rich foods, our bodies simply produce less cholesterol to compensate, so our overall blood cholesterol levels remain relatively constant.

Most of the cholesterol we eat in the Alkaline Life, including coconut oil, is in the form that means it is not absorbed by our body and is instead excreted by our gut.[62] So there's no cholesterol risk around consuming coconut oil.

We'll discuss this in more depth in Chapter 17, but for now I just want you to feel confident to eat these healthy fats.

The Best Fats: Omega-3 and Saturated Fats

The fats you'll be focusing on in the Alkaline Life are omega-3 and saturated fat from coconut oil.

Omega-3 is an essential fatty acid, meaning we *must* consume it, as the body cannot manufacture it. It's important in so many ways, and sadly, so many people are chronically deficient in it. A study out of the Harvard School of Public Health showed omega-3 deficiency to be the sixth biggest cause of preventable mortality in the United States.[63]

Why Are We So Deficient?

For most of the general public, fish is their only source of omega-3, and most people don't consume a lot of fish. The U.S. Department of Agriculture suggests that most people are consuming just less than one serving of seafood per week (including fish and shellfish). Without supplementing or consuming lots of the alkaline-forming, fat-rich foods we've already discussed, one would be considerably deficient in omega-3.

The second reason for this deficiency is the concerningly high levels of omega-6 and omega-9 in the SMD. Omega-6 is rampant in the SMD, as it is the main fat in cheap, processed vegetable and seed oils such as corn, canola, soybean, sunflower, safflower, and cottonseed oil. These oils are used in processed food and fast food, snack foods, and baked goods, and as a culture, we are massively overconsuming them. When omega-6 intake is high, it can interfere with the body's ability to absorb and utilize omega-3s, leading to an imbalance of these fatty acids in the body.

The ideal daily ratio of omega-3 to omega-6 we should be aiming for is 2:1, or even 1:1. However, estimates suggest that in the West, this ratio is closer to 1:20.

Too much omega-6 is pro-inflammatory, acidic, and causes considerable oxidative stress. We need to be mindful of the recommended ratios and eat consciously to get enough omega-3 into our diet.

We should be aiming for around 3 g of omega-3 per day, whether that's from eicosapentaenoic acid (EPA), docosahexaenoic acid (DHA), or alpha-linolenic acid (ALA). Ideally a mixture is good. There's some evidence to suggest that ALA is less potent, as it needs to be converted by the body to become usable. However, this process is quite simple, and this is still a very necessary and powerful fatty acid.

Saturated Fat

This is quite simple: eat lots of coconut! That's all there is to it! The benefits from the medium-chain triglycerides (MCTs) in coconut are incredible.

You want to aim to consume around a teaspoon to a tablespoon of coconut oil per day. You can cook with coconut oil and add it to smoothies, soups, porridge, and stews. You can take it straight from the spoon (if you're in a location where it's warm enough that the oil is liquid; I don't recommend doing this when it's solid!).

You can also get coconut fat via coconut cream and coconut milk, but they aren't something most people should consume enough of daily to make them a consistent source. See these as a bonus.

While there is an upper tolerable limit to saturated fat, plant-based saturated fats are quite easily absorbed, digested, and eliminated by the body,[64] so it can simply get rid of what it doesn't need. And with coconut as your primary source of saturated fat, you would need to eat a bizarre amount of coconut oil to cause yourself any concern.

While I am not saying you must reduce your saturated fat from dairy and meat to zero, plant-based saturated fats are more beneficial than saturated fats in meat or dairy. In a study published in *The BMJ*, coconut oil outperformed butter in both raising healthy HDL cholesterol and lowering the "bad" LDL cholesterol.[65] Again, I am not saying you have to avoid all animal sources of saturated fats, but the data I have seen shows plant-based is a better choice.

Coconut oil is also a potent anti-inflammatory, further strengthening its benefit for the cardiovascular system.[66]

Aside from the cardiovascular and cholesterol pieces, there are several other reasons why I want you to consume coconut oil daily:

- **Immune support.** Coconut oil contains lauric acid, which has been shown to have antimicrobial properties that can help protect against infections and support the immune system.[67]

- **Anti-Candida.** Caprylic acid, also found in coconut oil, is proven to destroy several strains of candida, including *Candida albicans*. When used both internally and topically against candida infections, it's incredibly potent. Consuming coconut oil is a great defense against candida overgrowth in the body.[68]

- **Energy boosting.** MCTs are easily digested by the body and do not require bile to break down, which means they're quickly converted to energy and don't need to be stored as fat. They're also absorbed quickly and easily and are transported directly to the liver, where they can be used for energy.[69]

- **Brain health.** The MCTs in coconut oil, particularly caprylic acid, have been studied extensively for their benefits to the brain. Studies have shown caprylic acid has cognitive benefits for people with Alzheimer's disease and other neurological disorders. Caprylic acid is thought to be particularly beneficial for the brain's health due to its ability to provide it with a quick source of energy. The brain is highly dependent on glucose for energy, and when glucose levels are low (such as during fasting or low-carb diets), it can use ketones, which are produced when the body breaks down fats. The liver can metabolize caprylic acid to make ketones for this alternative brain fuel source.[70]

Coconut Oil vs. MCT Oil

Coconut oil contains approximately 42 percent lauric acid, 7 percent caprylic acid, and 5 percent capric acid, as well as long-chain triglycerides (LCTs) and unsaturated fats. MCT oil is simply an *extract* of two of the fatty acids in coconut oil: C8, caprylic acid; and C10, capric acid.

The extract is available because some folks want the benefits of just those two fatty acids. And this is reasonable, as these are the fatty acids most associated with cognitive benefits and are the dominant fatty acids converted by the liver into ketones.

Rather than deciding which to use, I would use both. Coconut oil is better for cooking and does have the more rounded health profile, whereas MCT oil is totally flavorless and odorless and so can be taken from the spoon like a supplement while being much gentler on the gastrointestinal tract. For some people, coconut oil can cause a feeling of nausea or digestive issues, whereas MCT oil doesn't usually do this.

Phew! That was a bit about fats and oils! But I believe it was necessary. There are so many misperceptions out there about fats and oils, and you really need to jump in with both feet on this.

The Complete Guide to Healthy Fats and Oils

If you would like to get a full deep dive on fats, oils, optimizing cholesterol, and heart health, including the studies, uses, and ins and outs of good and bad fats, head to www.thealkalinelife book.com/fats to download my free 37-page guide.

ANTI-INFLAMMATORY FOODS

As we discussed, all alkaline-forming foods are naturally anti-inflammatory; however, there are two superpowerful anti-inflammatory foods that I want you to focus on including in your diet: turmeric and ginger.

The compound in turmeric called *curcumin* has been proven to be perhaps *the* most powerfully anti-inflammatory compound we know of. It has been studied in over 12,000 peer-reviewed and published biomedical papers and is *so* powerful that in studies, it outperforms several OTC medications for cholesterol optimization[71] in place of corticosteroids[72] and also in place of anti-inflammatory drugs such as aspirin and ibuprofen.[73]

Curcumin is so powerfully anti-inflammatory that I highly, highly recommend you consume it daily (I'll show you how in Part III).

If you have a specific inflammatory-based health challenge such as arthritis, fibromyalgia, polycystic ovary syndrome (PCOS), lupus, IBS or IBD, psoriasis, cardiovascular disease, type 2 diabetes, or any autoimmune disease, consuming curcumin daily is a must and will bring huge rewards.

But no matter who you are and what your health challenge is, inflammation in some form likely plays a role in preventing you from being where you want to be, and we need to address the issue.

Ginger contains several bioactive compounds, such as gingerols and shogaols, that have been shown to inhibit the production of pro-inflammatory molecules in the body, including cytokines and chemokines, and it contains compounds that can inhibit the activity of an enzyme called *cyclooxygenase-2* (COX-2), which plays a key role in the production of pro-inflammatory molecules.[74]

While not as powerful as turmeric, ginger is a close second, and it is, of course, delicious.

As you move through the steps of the plan in Part III, you'll see how effortlessly we get turmeric and ginger into your everyday life. You can add it to juices and smoothies, grate it into salads, include it in stir-fries, and blend it into soups and stews. We enjoy turmeric and ginger teas and lattes, and we roast our veggies in them too.

Anti-inflammatory foods to focus on: turmeric, ginger, asparagus, bell pepper, avocado, beet, garlic, onion, cruciferous vegetables, and leafy greens.

ALKALINE PROTEIN-RICH FOODS

Protein is something people get overly worried about. Whether it's living alkaline or simply going vegan or vegetarian, we've all been asked the question a million times over: "But where do you get your protein?"

I'm not sure why people believe that the only sources of protein are meat and dairy, but rest assured, you'll be consuming plenty enough protein in the Alkaline Life Plan. Dependent on your goal, you may want to specifically include more protein in your diet, but most people will not need to give it a second thought, because they will already be getting lots.

If you want to add more, this is awesome too! Whether it's for a specific health challenge or because you're doing a lot of resistance training and looking to build muscle mass, getting enough protein while eating alkaline is quite easy.

Protein is, of course, essential for so many functions and processes in the body. We absolutely need it. But we don't need *masses* of it, and we can get it from plenty of different sources.

Here are some of my favorite sources of alkaline protein:

Lentils and beans: up to 19.7 g per cup
Chia seeds: 17.1 g per 100 g
Oats: 26.4 g per cup
Raw, alkaline protein powder: approximately 70 g per 100 g
    (around 20 to 25 g per serving)
Quinoa: 9.1 g per cup

Nuts and seeds: up to 29.8 g per 100 g
Nut butter: 18 g per 100 g
Tofu: 32 g per 100 g

If you want to go a little further and include a protein supplement, you can certainly do so if you need it for your exercise or health goal. I give my recommendations on protein supplements in Chapter 7.

High-protein foods to focus on: lentils, beans, oats, chia and other seeds, quinoa, nuts, tofu, edamame, leafy greens, broccoli, nut milks, and nut butters.

A Typical Day on the Alkaline Life Plan

Using the recipes in this book, your typical day of living the Alkaline Life could look like this:

Pre-Breakfast: Creamy Turmeric & Ginger Warmer Tea: protein—2.6 g; 17 oz lemon water: protein—0 g

Breakfast: Alkaline All-Day Energy Smoothie: protein—22 g; Alkaline Oats: protein—18 g

Snack: Nut & Seed Mix: protein—19 g

Lunch: Quinoa & Hummus Wraps: protein—18.9 g

Snack: Celery Sticks with Almond Butter: protein—7.9 g

Dinner: Alkaline Thai Green Curry with Brown Rice—protein 54 g

Total protein intake: 142 g

This is without the use of supplements. A scoop of alkaline protein powder would add another 25 grams of protein to this, to take it to 167 grams.

Protein Quantity vs. Quality

We should quickly note that the sheer number of protein grams consumed per day is not actually the most important measure. The amino acid consumption, which is a big indicator of the protein *quality*, is just as important, if not more.

Again, applying 20/80, three amino acids are probably more important than the others combined: lysine, leucine, and methionine.

These three amino acids are abundant in nuts, seeds, and beans. So if you're concerned about protein, make sure you focus on quality as much as quantity.

LOW-SUGAR FRUITS

The question of fruits is such an important one to understand when you're first starting on the Alkaline Life. Not all fruits are created equal, and while there are a lot of fruits you can eat with wild abandon, it's a mistake to think that all fruits are alkaline forming. You can easily fall into the trap of overconsuming them. Yes, you can overconsume certain fruits. But I want you to understand that *I am not, in any way, saying you should not eat fruit.*

Fruit is a fantastic source of so many vitamins and minerals. However, you should ideally aim to stick to the lower-sugar fruits, primarily berries, and see the higher-sugar fruits (banana, pineapple, orange, apple) as treats.

But to keep this totally real, a high-sugar fruit like a banana, while acid forming, is *far* healthier than a chocolate bar! So don't stress too much about fruits. Eat the lower-sugar fruits as much as you like and keep the higher sugar fruits to 1 to 2 servings per day.

Fructose Is the Issue

Fruit, as delicious as it is, contains fructose. And fructose is a problem. While most types of sugar can be metabolized by practically every cell in the body, fructose can be metabolized *only* by the liver. We were not designed to eat the vast volumes of fructose that we do today. Regular sugars—table sugar, brown sugar, raw sugar, cane sugar—these are all 50 percent glucose and 50 percent fructose. Don't get me wrong; the glucose *is* acidic, oxidizing, inflammatory, and bad news—but if you're moderately active, the body can use it.

Fructose cannot be used, and it stresses the heck out of the liver, the pancreas, and so much more.

People think of fructose as a "natural" sugar, "fruit" sugar, or "healthy" sugar, but this is just not the case. It's not only as damaging as any other sugar; in reality, it's actually worse.

Fructose metabolism causes inflammation, liver stress, oxidative stress, and uric acid formation, and it makes us gain weight, because it makes us want to keep eating more.

Now, that's not to say that fruit is the *biggest* source of fructose we're eating. That award is comfortably taken by high-fructose corn syrup in processed foods. However, I strongly recommend you don't juice, blend, or dehydrate fruits. Eat them whole and raw.

Fructose is far less damaging when consumed with fiber and chewed and digested slowly. When the fiber is removed (as with juices), it's more rapidly metabolized by the liver. Same goes for dried fruits. These give a huge hit of fructose with very little fiber and immediately stress the liver.

So there should be no fruit in juices (because the fiber is removed) or even in smoothies, because if your smoothie contains several servings of fruit and you drink the smoothie at a normal pace, this overloads the liver very quickly (think about the time it takes to drink a drink versus to eat two to three pieces of fruit, including chewing time).

The least acid-forming, lowest fructose-containing fruits are berries, and my personal favorite is blueberries. Packed with nutrients and antioxidants, blueberries are fantastic for the brain, eyes, immune system,[75] and heart.[76]

Fruits to focus on: blueberries, strawberries, grapefruit, watermelon, raspberries, blackberries, papaya, and kiwi.

THE MOST IMPORTANT ALKALINE FOODS TO FOCUS ON

Leafy greens, nuts, seeds, cruciferous vegetables, fruits, oily fish, lentils, beans, herbs, and spices: you can see how living the Alkaline Life is full of wonderfully varied, delicious foods, *plus* there's room for you to still include that 20 percent or so of some meat, a little of the right dairy, a glass of red wine, and so on.

But it's not all sunshine, butterflies, and rainbows. There are some seriously acid-forming foods we need to talk about. Some can be kept in your 20 percent "treat" bucket and used here and there alongside the alkaline foods. Others need to be kept for a *real* treat moment. And some need to be removed completely.

It's important to note that you don't have to stress about *any* of them on day one. We'll move slowly, day by day, to where we want to be—one step at a time. And I'll show you how to make it easy and sustainable for your everyday life in Part III.

Ali's Story

I started on the alkaline journey because of a brain tumor diagnosis (oligodendroglioma).

I had brain surgery, chemo, and radiation and was exhausted every day. My weight was the highest it had ever been in my life. I was running on fumes, needing multiple cups of coffee and energy drinks all day just to function. I just felt terrible.

Since then, I'm thrilled to report the tumor has disappeared, and I have lost over 50 pounds [23 kilograms].

My blood tests are now all at healthy levels: total cholesterol from 208 to 153, LDL from 132 to 77, and triglycerides went from 222 all the way down to 34!

With living the Alkaline Life, my energy is at an all-time high, and all without the need for caffeine. I feel better than I've ever felt before.

CHAPTER 5

Acidic Offenders: The Foods You Should Steer Clear Of

This is the chapter you might have been dreading. But before we jump into foods to avoid, I want you to remember that you don't have to give up anything forever, and there's lots of wiggle room in the Alkaline Life for treats and cheat meals. I want to put your mind at ease and reiterate: the goal is not perfection. The goal is to have balance.

Once we start getting into these acid-forming foods, I also want you to remember that there's a sliding scale of how acid forming they are. Some are mildly so, and others are best to limit to rare treats.

You'll also probably find, like most of my Alkaline Life Club members, that a lot of the foods on the acidic list are things you can simply live without and that have been in your diet only because of old habits and routine.

With the simple strategies I'll share in Part III, there are no acid-forming foods that we don't have a delicious, simple alternative for. It won't be scary, so let's get into it.

SUGAR AND SWEETENERS

The combination of a lack of healthy fat in the diet and a dramatic increase in sugar intake is devastating. Sugar is killing us, straight up. We are eating so much more than we need to, and it's destroying our health.

Sugar is added to *everything* nowadays, and we're consuming a *lot* more processed and packaged foods than ever before. Not only are we time poor, busy, and reaching for convenience more than ever, but Big Food has worked out how to make these products cheap, easy, and highly addictive.

We've all seen the studies showing how sugar can be as addictive as cocaine,[1] but on top of this, Big Food is so clever at developing flavor, texture, and ingredient combinations to make products that are irresistible. Unless we find ways to cut them out, how can we win?

In 2022 the average person in the United States was consuming 126.4 grams of sugar per day.[2] The American Heart Association recommends 24 grams per day for women and 36 grams for men.[3] Every *day* we are consuming 425 percent more than is safe for women and 250 percent more than is safe for men.

Overconsumption of sugar is a huge contributor to type 2 diabetes,[4] obesity,[5] heart disease,[6] cancer,[7] liver disease,[8] and Alzheimer's.[9] But nobody is telling us to quit. Foods don't come with warning labels, and no governments are removing sugar from their "healthy" eating guides.

All of this is to say that it's not your fault. The odds have been stacked against you. Sugar has been hidden everywhere and added to everything. Seemingly harmless foods are actually addictive sugar bombs, and nobody is telling you to stop eating it!

How Much Sugar Is in Your Diet?

Most people are surprised when they calculate how much sugar they consume on an average day. Look at this quite typical day of someone who probably believes they're following a "healthy" diet:

Breakfast

> Orange juice (1 cup)
> Raisin bran (1 cup)
> Low-fat milk (½ cup)

Midmorning Snack

> Blueberry yogurt (1 cup)

Lunch

> Apple juice (1 cup)
> Cheese sandwich
> Peach

Midafternoon Snack

> Frozen yogurt smoothie (16 ounces)

Dinner

> Pizza (1 slice)
> Salad with store-bought dressing
> Soda (1 can)

It might surprise you that the person eating this has consumed 295 grams of sugar. How can that even happen? Let's look at each of these foods with their sugar content:

- Orange juice (1 cup) – 28 g / 7 teaspoons
- Raisin bran (1 cup) – 20 g / 5 teaspoons
- Low-fat milk (½ cup) – 6 g / 1 teaspoon
- Blueberry yogurt (1 cup) – 24 g / 6 teaspoons
- Apple juice (1 cup) – 40 g / 10 teaspoons
- Cheese sandwich – 6 g / 1 teaspoon
- Peach – 9 g / 2 teaspoons
- Frozen yogurt smoothie (16 oz) – 94 g / 23 teaspoons

- Pizza (1 slice) – 4 g / 1 teaspoon
- Salad with store-bought dressing – 12 g / 3 teaspoons
- Soda (12 oz) – 52 g / 13 teaspoons

Total sugars for the day: 295 g / 72 teaspoons

Of course, there are some obvious offenders, but even if we take out the smoothie and soda, we're looking at 149 grams for the day. This is still six times higher than the recommendation.

I cannot stress this enough: it is *essential* that your sugar intake is lower than the recommended maximum of 50 grams per day. This is your first step with sugar, and following the steps in this book will make that a breeze.

The next step is to average 25 to 35 grams per day as a maximum. This is achievable, especially when you consider that most of the sugar in the average diet consists of *added* sugar, not the small number of natural sugars present in the fresh vegetables and whole fruits you'll be eating. And 25 to 35 grams *does* leave room for some treats. If you're a bit over some days because you've had a date night, this is totally awesome. So don't stress. Just follow the steps in Part III.

The Great Sugar Swap

A fast and powerful tool I developed for you to get your sugar consumption down 80 percent without any hard work or sacrifice is called the "Great Sugar Swap." To download this tool, head to www.thealkalinelifebook.com/sugar.

Sweeteners

Just, no. Sweeteners, including aspartame, saccharin, and sucralose are incredibly toxic, carcinogenic, acidic, hormone-disrupting, gut-flora-destroying, inflammatory nightmares. Please, simply do not eat these. Many studies have linked them to cancer,[10] weight gain,[11] insulin resistance,[12] and cardiovascular disease.[13] A 2010 study also linked artificial sweetener use with an increased risk of miscarriage and preterm birth. They're toxic chemicals that have no right to be in your body.

Ditch them now.

The only argument is for their "zero-calorie" status, but even if you believe that calories in versus calories out is the way to lose weight (we discuss this in Chapter 10), all of the data tells us that long-term sweetener use is linked to weight gain and an increased risk of type 2 diabetes.

Natural Sugars

Sugars that are still in their natural state (such as in a piece of whole fruit) are fine. The problem is when humankind has meddled with them, refined them, and made them into something else. As we discussed, fructose, when concentrated, is a huge issue. When processed by the liver, it is pro-inflammatory, acidic, and hormone disrupting, creating excess fat cells and excess insulin.

When you remember that most sugars and syrups—including honey, maple syrup, date syrup, coconut syrup and sugar, and so on—are up to 50 percent fructose, you can see why these are not the best choice.

The Good Alternative

I have a couple of recommendations for you:

> *Instead of syrups*: use rice malt syrup (sometimes called brown rice syrup). It is not alkaline forming by any means, but it is a better alternative, as it does not contain fructose.
>
> *Instead of sugars*: use stevia. Avoid xylitol, as it is highly refined and quite pro-inflammatory.* [14]

---

* There's been a recent study linking erythritol to heart disease, but the findings are not quite what some people have suggested. It's important to note that the subjects of the study were all very sick. Over 70 percent had hypertension, over 40 percent had already had at least one heart attack, 75 percent had arterial disease, and 25 percent had type 2 diabetes—and the study was looking at blood levels of erythritol, not erythritol intake. These findings cannot be extrapolated to say erythritol causes heart disease. However, it is more highly processed, so my advice is to stick to stevia if you need to add a sweetener.

Honey, particularly manuka honey, can be used in moderation for its antiviral properties, but don't consume it as a daily food.

GLUTEN

If sugar is *the* most acidic substance on earth, gluten is a close second. In fact, I'm going to say they are equal first on a practical level. We absolutely need to get gluten out of our diet.

It is incredibly acid forming and possibly even more pro-inflammatory than sugar. Many people do not realize quite how devastating gluten is for your endocrine system and all of the hormones it manages, particularly regarding spiking insulin levels.

Most gluten you consume is in gluten-containing grains like wheat, rye, and spelt products, and while there is a little hidden elsewhere in the diet (in soy sauce, for example), don't worry too much about the little details. Just look to swap out the big offenders: bread, cereals, pasta, couscous, noodles, baked goods, and pastries. I know for a lot of people, the thought of giving these up is a scary one, but as you'll see in Part III, it's actually quite straightforward, and I promise that you will not miss these foods at all.

Like sugar, there are myriad ways that gluten is damaging to your health. And like sugar, gluten can be quite addictive. If you've ever felt like you're addicted to bread and pasta, it's possible you are! Research has suggested that gluten-containing foods may impact the brain's reward system by triggering the release of dopamine, a neurotransmitter associated with feelings of pleasure and satisfaction. This release of dopamine may lead some people to feel a sense of euphoria or a "high" when consuming gluten-containing foods, which can create a desire for more.[15]

So again, if you've been consuming a lot of gluten and sugar, it's not your fault!

However, we need to cut it back immediately, and ideally eliminate it, over time—completely.

Here are just a handful of problems with consuming gluten.

Insulin Resistance

Consuming gluten spikes blood sugar like nothing else. Remember, insulin resistance is the condition in which the body's cells become less responsive to insulin, a hormone produced by the pancreas to help regulate blood sugar levels. The more we spike blood sugars, the more insulin we produce, and the less sensitive the body becomes to it. This means the body has to produce more and more to create the same impact, leading to higher levels of insulin in the bloodstream. Over time, this can lead to a range of complications, including type 2 diabetes, obesity, high blood pressure, and heart disease.

Gluten is especially dangerous when it comes to insulin resistance, because it contains a supercarbohydrate called *amylopectin-A*.

While gluten-containing products have a high glycemic index, meaning they are quickly absorbed and digested and create a rapid spike in blood sugar levels, there are three more nefarious ways that amylopectin-A can quickly cause insulin resistance.[16] They are:

1. *Inflammation.* Amylopectin-A has been shown to stimulate the production of pro-inflammatory cytokines,[17] which can contribute to the development of insulin resistance. Chronic inflammation in the body can impair the function of insulin-producing cells in the pancreas, as well as the insulin-sensitive cells in the liver, muscle, and fat tissues.[18]

2. *Oxidative stress.* High levels of blood sugar, particularly when they occur frequently and repeatedly, can lead to oxidative stress in the body. This can damage cells and tissues and impair their function, leading to the development of insulin resistance.[19]

3. *Increased fat accumulation.* Some studies have suggested that a diet high in amylopectin-A may lead to increased fat accumulation in the liver and other organs.[20] This can lead to impaired insulin signaling and contribute to the development of insulin resistance.[21]

Of course, we want to avoid insulin resistance at all costs!

Inflammation

When we consume gluten, it triggers an immune response in the gut, leading to the release of inflammatory cytokines and the activation of immune cells. This gut imbalance leads to a cascade of other issues.

We also know that the release of the cytokines interleukin-1 (IL-1), interleukin-6 (IL-6), and tumor necrosis factor alpha cause the body to create and store fat cells that then produce a vicious cycle of more and more inflammation.

It is all linked and becomes a complex web, but eliminating gluten and including super-nourishing, delicious, anti-inflammatory, alkaline-forming foods into your diet can help undo this damage.

Leaky Gut (Intestinal Permeability)

Leaky gut refers to a condition in which the lining of the small intestine becomes more porous than normal, allowing potentially harmful substances to enter the bloodstream. Gluten is perhaps *the* biggest dietary contributor to leaky gut. When we consume it, it activates a protein called *zonulin*, which opens the tight junctures of the gut wall, creating lots of little holes that allow the entry of undigested matter and toxins into the bloodstream.

This is one of the biggest triggers of autoimmune conditions, as the immune system tries over and over to attack these particles that have reentered the bloodstream.

Hormone Disruption

Consuming gluten can trigger the body's immune system to mistakenly attack the thyroid gland, causing inflammation and damage.

In addition to these autoimmune responses, gluten may also interfere with the absorption of important nutrients that are needed for thyroid function, such as selenium and zinc.

The bottom line is, we need to eliminate gluten. We'll do this gently and over time in the Alkaline Life Plan in Part III. For now, to make sure we're on the same page as to which grains contain gluten and which do not, here's a list.

Grains to Reduce or Avoid

- Wheat
- Rye
- Spelt
- Barley
- Bulgur

The "grains" and other products that people often *think* contain gluten but are absolutely fine to include are:

Grains That Are Allowed

- Rice
- Quinoa
- Buckwheat
- Amaranth
- Millet
- Sorghum
- Teff
- Oats (if certified gluten-free)

Plus, the following products are gluten-free:

- Coconut flour
- Almond flour
- Chickpea flour
- Tapioca flour/starch
- Potato starch
- Arrowroot
- Flaxseed meal
- Chia seeds

Oats are often a confusing one, because people see a label that says "gluten-free" oats, and they assume that oats generally contain gluten. However, oats are naturally gluten-free. The reason that oats are labeled "gluten-free" is that most are milled in facilities that also produce wheat, rye, and so on, and the risk of contamination could be enough to trigger a reaction in those who are hypersensitive. "Gluten-free" oats are made in a certified gluten-free facility. If you are not a hypersensitive celiac, you can eat regular oats but may still choose the gluten-free variety when available.

ANIMAL PROTEIN

Meat is highly acidic and requires a lot of energy to break down. The digestion of meat, and the sulfur and phosphorus in its proteins, leads to the production of excessive sulfuric and phosphoric acid as well as a huge spike in uric acid, all of which are hugely taxing to the body's alkaline buffering system.[22] But while no animal protein is alkaline forming, there is a difference between cheap, mass-produced meat and ethically raised, organic, grass-fed meat.

Please don't mistake this for me saying you can eat as much grass-fed steak as you want. Meat is still acid forming, but if you want to include it in your 20 percent, then I'm not going to tell you that you can't. You should just focus on high-quality meats as much as you possibly can.

The Type of Meat You Must Avoid

For all the acid-forming impacts of consuming meat, *processed* meat is 10 times worse. It is almost a whole other food. The preservatives and chemicals used in the processing of bacon, sausages, deli meats, and hot dogs are hugely acidic and pro-inflammatory.

One of the most significant health risks associated with processed meat is an increased risk of cancer. The International Agency for Research on Cancer has classified processed meat as a Group 1 carcinogen, meaning that there is strong evidence linking its consumption to an increased risk of colorectal cancer.[23] Other types of cancer, such as stomach and pancreatic cancer, have also been associated with the consumption of processed meat.[24]

The nitrates used in processed meat are also strongly linked with increased type 2 diabetes[25] risk, neurodegenerative disorders,[26] and heart disease.[27] They cause massive inflammation and oxidative stress and are of course highly acid forming.

Can I Still Eat Meat and Live Alkaline?

Meat is acid forming. But as you know, you don't have to be *perfect* to live the Alkaline Life. Many of my Alkaline Life Club members still eat meat as part of their diet and are thriving, and while I don't personally, I would never say you cannot. There are, however, a few recommended rules to make sure you get the most out of this.

1. Eat meat 2 to 3 times per week maximum, such that you look forward to the occasion.
2. Aim for the most ethically farmed/raised product. Not only is this kinder to the animal and better for the environment, but ethically raised animals tend to be the most healthily raised and fed.
3. Spend your usual weekly budget for meat, but only on the very best quality you can find. Buy direct from trusted farms if possible. Not only will this raise the quality of what you eat, but it will reduce the quantity too! Grass-fed provides nutrient-dense protein, while grain-fed is nutrient poor.

DAIRY

The average U.S. adult consumes around 628 pounds of dairy per year, including milk, ice cream, cheese, and yogurt.[28] Yet it is an acidic, mucus-producing, sugar-laden, hormone-and-chemical-heavy, pro-inflammatory food we can easily eliminate.

There is no nutrient in dairy that we cannot easily get elsewhere in our diet, and in ways that contribute to our vitality rather than reduce it.

I know, I know, *we've been told for decades that dairy is good for our bones.*

But it's not completely true. There are two factors here that are essential to understand as to why we've been told this (and continue to be):

1. It's worth billions of dollars to the dairy industry worldwide if we keep believing this myth, so they fund research, launch advertising campaigns, lobby governments, and make very generous donations where necessary.

2. The logic is based on the pure calcium content of dairy products.

The notion that dairy contains calcium and therefore strengthens our bones is incredibly simplistic and ignores the other components in milk and dairy, such as lactose and D-galactose, that create a net calcium *loss* in the body.

While it is true that dairy is high in calcium, the effect of the lactose, D-galactose, and other unhealthy sugars overpowers the net intake of calcium. Dairy is strongly acid forming, and as we've discussed, when the body must buffer acidity, it draws minerals from the bones and other areas to help neutralize it. The bones *lose* more calcium due to these sugars and other toxins than they gain from the calcium that can be absorbed from the milk.

Additional Problems with Dairy

Dairy has been linked to increased risk of cardiovascular disease,[29] cancer[30] (particularly prostate cancer[31]), asthma,[32] and, of course, osteoporosis.[33, 34, 35] Plus, the sugars lactose, and D-galactose are linked to insulin resistance,[36] and more.

Got Calcium?

Calcium is incredibly important, but dairy is not a good way to get it into the diet. If you're concerned about getting enough, there are plenty of amazing alkaline-forming, plant-based sources of calcium. Considering that a half-cup serving of full-fat milk contains 113 milligrams of calcium, you don't need to go too far to see there are better alternatives per serving:

- Almonds: 264 mg
- Bok choy: 37 mg

- Broccoli: 47 mg
- Chia seeds: 631 mg
- Collard greens: 232 mg
- Edamame: 60 mg
- Hazelnuts: 114 mg
- Kale: 47 mg
- Mustard greens: 115 mg
- Navy beans: 127 mg
- Quinoa: 31 mg
- Sesame seeds: 975 mg
- Spinach: 99 mg
- Sunflower seeds: 78 mg
- Tofu: 200 mg
- Turnip greens: 190 mg

BAD "FATS"

Bad fats are flat-out toxic. But I honestly wish they weren't called fats. It gives good fats a bad name.

When we're talking about "bad" fats, we're talking trans fats, hydrogenated, and semi- or partially hydrogenated fats, as well as cheap vegetable oils.

Trans fats are artificially produced, created by adding hydrogen to liquid vegetable oils. They are commonly found in processed foods such as fried foods, baked goods, and snacks like chips and crackers. Trans fats can increase LDL (bad) cholesterol levels and decrease HDL (good) cholesterol levels, which can increase the risk of heart disease and stroke.

Highly processed vegetable oils such as corn oil, soybean oil, and canola oil are commonly used in processed foods, fast foods, and fried foods. A lot of the problems associated with these bad fats are associated with their super-high omega-6 content. And while there is benefit to having a *little* omega-6 in the diet from healthy, plant-based sources such as nuts and seeds, the catastrophically huge volumes of omega-6 that are in the SMD from these processed vegetable oils and all of the processed foods we're now eating is, frankly, dangerous.

When omega-6 is consumed in excess, it's strongly correlated with an increased risk of oxidative stress,[37] autoimmune issues,[38] diabetes,[39] heart disease,[4·] cancer,[41] and obesity.[42] Remember, we're designed to consume an omega-3-to-omega-6 ratio of around 2:1, but we're actually now consuming a ratio of close to 1:20 or more.[43]

Margarine

Everything I've just said for those oils goes tenfold for margarine. In addition, margarine contains highly carcinogenic, hormone-disrupting chemicals, artificial colors and flavors, and preservatives that just throw more fuel onto the inflammatory fire. Its fats are meant to be liquid, and they're meant to be clear. To turn them into a spreadable solid that is "yellow" like butter . . . let's just say your health is not the most important consideration here.

The Worst of the Rest! Other Acid-Forming Foods to Limit

We've covered the big picture that accounts for 95 percent or more of the acid-forming foods that appear in most people's lives. But there are a few others that don't really fit these categories, or are the random, little ingredients that people ask about all the time. So let's quickly cover some of these now.

Caffeine. When we consume caffeine, the adrenals produce and release cortisol, driving down our blood pH. Over time, this can also impact adrenal function, leading to adrenal fatigue and the various health challenges that can come from this. A cup of coffee here and there is not an issue, but consuming coffee daily or multiple times per day is definitely not recommended.

Apple cider vinegar (ACV). While ACV is a "healthier" vinegar than most, it is most definitely acid forming. Despite what some people have claimed, ACV is not alkaline forming once digested, primarily because it contains acetic acid, which unbalances gut flora and requires significant buffering to neutralize. If you have any digestive issues or if your health challenges are rooted in digestive imbalance (including fatigue, weight, reflux, gout, inflammation, and so on), please steer clear of ACV. It's fine to use in a recipe here and there, but it shouldn't be used daily or as a supplement.

Nutritional yeast. Yeast is 100 percent acid forming. Adding it to food is not a good idea, and definitely do not use it as a supplement.

Sourdough bread. I get asked about sourdough a lot, and while it's far less processed than other breads, it's still made with gluten-containing grains.

Fermented foods. Sauerkraut, kimchi, kombucha, miso, and so on are not to be seen as health foods or consumed regularly. They are fine treats to be used here and there, but they're quite acid forming. If you need to rebalance gut bacteria, I recommend my Weed, Seed, Feed protocol (page 132).

Mushrooms. All mushrooms are acid forming. *But there is a caveat.* Some mushrooms do have potent health benefits for very specific conditions. If you're under the guidance of a Traditional Chinese Medicine practitioner, use the herbs and mushrooms they prescribe for the set period they give you.

Bone broth. Bone broth is actually fine to use! The acid-forming nature of the animal protein is heavily offset by the concentrated minerals in the broth. You can absolutely continue to use bone broth, and collagen supplements too.

Remember, you can get my Definitive Acid/Alkaline Food Chart with over 400 foods ranked at www.thealkalinelifebook.com.

CHAPTER 6

You Are What You Drink, So Don't Drink Acid!

You can eat perfectly alkaline but still end up acidic if you don't watch what you drink. Beverages can be a sneaky way for a huge volume of acidity entering into your body. Hydration is key. It's important that you consume the right liquids, so that what you drink *contributes* to your health instead of takes away from it.

ACID- AND ALKALINE-FORMING DRINKS

We need to make sure our drinks are contributing to, and not removing from, our health. It's great to be eating lots of greens, healthy fats, turmeric, and veggies, but if we are then drinking several cups of coffee, soda, and a bottle of wine, it more than undoes all of our hard work.

Again, there's always room for treats, but day-to-day, you need to be making the smarter choice.

The most acid-forming drinks that appear most commonly in the SMD are:

- Soda
- Cordial
- Fruit juices
- Coffee and tea
- Alcohol
- Carbonated water (which is acidic, due to the carbonic acid content)
- Iced teas, "vitamin drinks," and other "healthy" store-bought beverages.

None of these should be a surprise. Some wonder whether fruit juice is healthy, but it absolutely isn't and should be avoided. The concentrated fructose (and fruit juice can contain more sugar than soda) is terribly acidic and inflammatory.

THE ALKALINE DRINKS TO FOCUS ON

Healthy hydration does not mean only water! While you should be consuming lots of clean, filtered water throughout the day, other options can include the following:

Herbal Tea

Noncaffeinated herbal tea is a great way to increase your daily hydration. My personal favorites include lemon and ginger, turmeric, ginger, mint, echinacea, hibiscus, passionflower, and rooibos. These are all noncaffeinated and full of antioxidants. Just 2 to 3 cups per day can add 30 ounces or more to your hydration.

While matcha and green tea do contain caffeine, you can still enjoy them in moderation. High-quality matcha contains a compound called *L-theanine*, which is useful, as it reduces the impact of the caffeine considerably and has a calming effect on the adrenals.[1]

Flavored Water

Another great choice to make your hydration more exciting than simple water is to add natural flavor to it. These days, lots of people are on board with drinking lemon water in the morning, but let's get more creative than that!

I absolutely love to make a big jug of water flavored with all sorts of fruits, herbs, veggies, and spices to drink throughout the morning. It's an idea that came about in our house due to our football (aka soccer)-obsessed kids. Football in Australia is somewhat hotter and more dehydrating than back in the U.K. Think sunburn and heatstroke being the concerns instead of muddy boots. While our kids' teammates seemed to be downing never-ending supplies of bright red sports drinks, we always felt a bit bad giving our boys plain water. So we started experimenting, and these infusions hit the spot! The beauty of it is that the kids really get involved in making funky flavors and trying new things.

Some of the favorites in our house are:

- Orange and blueberry
- Apple and cinnamon
- Apple and ginger
- Watermelon and mint
- Strawberry and basil
- Lemon and rosemary
- Rock melon (cantaloupe) and ginger
- Cucumber and lime
- Cucumber, mint, and lemon

All you need to do is chop up a bit of the fruit and throw it in with some of the torn herb, bash it about a bit, and you have a delicious infusion! Note that the amount of fructose in a bit of chopped fruit, such as 1 to 2 strawberries, is very different compared to the fructose from juicing a whole pineapple. There's no fructose worry with these concoctions!

Green Drinks

Juiced or powdered, green drinks are delicious and a great way to get super-nutrient-dense hydration into your day. A juice with celery, cucumber, spinach, kale, lettuce, turmeric, and ginger, watered down to taste, is perhaps the best alkaline-forming, electrolyte-rich hydration on earth.

Green *powders* are a fantastic supplement made from powdered grasses, green vegetables, herbs, spices, and low-sugar fruits. A scoop in a large glass of water is another incredible way to hydrate. I have had clients in the Alkaline Life Club achieve their first set of goals simply by adding 80 to 100 ounces of water with powdered greens to their daily life (it's a good example of 20/80).

I will explain more about these powders in Chapter 7, including the things to look for and avoid in a green powder, to help you add these to your daily life in a sustainable way.

THE BASICS OF ALKALINE WATER AND FILTERS

The most important thing to keep in mind about water is filtration. Tap water is frankly not acceptable. Between the chlorine, chloramines, fluoride, disinfectant by-products, agricultural runoff, and chemical spills, it is safe to say your tap water is sadly not a great choice.

Here are just a few headlines from the past couple of years:

- "Chlorine in Water Increases Birth Defects"[2]
- "Chemicals in Tap Water Could Cause 100,000 Cases of Cancer in U.S."[3]
- "Cancer Alert over South Australia's Tap Water"[4]
- "West Virginia Chemical Spill Triggers Tap Water Ban"[5]
- "Brain-Eating Amoeba in Tap Water Killed Child, Study Confirms"[6]
- "Lead in School Water Persists in US Despite Work to Fix the Problem. What Can Be Done?"[7]

- "Toxic Arsenic Levels Make Tap Water Unsafe for Thousands in New York City"[8]
- "Dangerous Arsenic Levels Found in Tap Water at Manhattan NYCHA Complex"[9]

These headlines are from national newspapers in the U.K., U.S., Canada, and Australia. And there are so many more. A three-year study by the Environmental Working Group (EWG) assembled an unprecedented database of 20 million drinking water quality tests performed by water utilities since 2004 and found 316 contaminants in U.S. tap water.[10] Among the contaminants were 202 chemicals that are not subject to any government regulation or safety standards for drinking water. That means they can just exist in our water at any level without needing to be tested for, screened for, or filtered out. If they're in there? Tough luck.

It's essential that you get some form of filtration for your tap water.

Whether it's a three-stage, under-sink, triple-cartridge filter system or a simple countertop jug, just get started. Don't get bogged down in the details.

The only water systems I do *not* recommend are reverse osmosis and distillers, as they both produce acid-forming water devoid of the natural minerals and water molecule structure your body craves. If you already have a reverse osmosis system, don't fear; you can remedy it to a certain degree by adding a remineralization canister to your setup for under $100.

If you want to take it further and get the full rundown on pH drops, alkaline water ionizers, hydrogen filters, and every other method of making alkaline water, I go through each in detail at wwww.thealkalinelifebook.com/water.

Is Bottled Water the Answer?

On the go, bottled water is fine. But you're better off using tap water instead of bottled water, and that's saying something. Bottled water is either from the same sources as tap water but without the testing and treating, or it's reverse-osmosis filtered. I've tested over 40 brands of bottled water, and each has been acid forming and oxidative-stress causing.

As for the so-called *alkaline* bottled water, this is just bottled water with a pinch of minerals added. None tested as any more alkaline than most tap waters.

That being said, I do want to emphasize that *proper hydration is absolutely essential.* If you're getting started right now, while you're still reading this book, please start drinking more water now!

Being hydrated is always far better than being dehydrated, even if it is with tap or bottled water. Your body can handle toxins just fine in moderation, so don't allow yourself to be dehydrated because you don't have access to a filter. Staying hydrated is absolutely essential. Just make sure you are not working against your health and drinking glass after glass of unfiltered water daily.

· CHAPTER 7 ·

The Alkaline Kitchen

I like to keep things simple. When it comes to the kitchen equipment you need, while having a great set of knives and all the gadgets is great, there are only two essentials. Then there are a few things that are nice to have.

A JUICER AND BLENDER ARE THE ONLY ESSENTIALS

For a juicer, I recommend getting an upright, cold-press juicer. The brand I absolutely love is Hurom. Its machines are incredibly powerful and reliable, and most important, so easy to clean. The cleanup process is a simple rinse. I have seen over the last two decades that what stops my clients from juicing, more than anything, is the unenjoyable cleanup at the end. With the Hurom juicers, there's no grate or grill to scrub, and the pulp doesn't get stuck in hard-to-reach places. It really is a 10-second rinse, and you're done.

I prefer the cold-press, masticating juicers that have a gear that slowly and gently squeezes the nutrients out of the food. The process of extracting the juice with a centrifugal juicer that whizzes and slices and grates the food at high speed is far more damaging to the nutrients and creates far more waste.

If you have a centrifugal juicer right now, don't worry; they're still great—but put a new cold-press juicer on your wish list!

For a blender, there are roughly two options: a cheap one or a not-so-cheap one! They all blend and smoothie foods, but the cheaper options have less power and can't easily handle ingredients like nuts, carrots, and beets. You won't get such a smooth consistency, and the cheaper blenders can burn out quite easily.

My personal preference is a Vitamix. They are so reliable and powerful, and I adore mine.

Do I Really Need a Juicer and a Blender?

Yes. Juicers make juice. Blenders make smoothies. You need both. You want to not only get the different benefits that juices and smoothies provide, but each also allows you to use quite different ingredients (you wouldn't, say, juice an avocado or blend celery). This is essential for getting the full *range* of nutrients.

While you theoretically can blend a lot of the juice recipes and then strain them with a cheesecloth to remove the fiber, this is simply a pain in the you-know-what, and it's critical to remove all annoying obstacles to making juicing a daily habit.

Juices and smoothies are *both* incredibly beneficial. I never recommend one over the other, and I do love to have them both. They do have differences, and there are strengths each has that make it "better" than the other, depending.

Difference #1: The Fiber

The biggest difference is that juice does not contain fiber. This is both a good thing *and* a bad thing.

It's a benefit not to contain fiber, because this means the nutrients can be much more efficiently and quickly delivered to your cells and everywhere they're needed in the body.

However, of course, this means *you're not getting the fiber!*

And one of the benefits of smoothies is that they *do* contain fiber—which is so important for your digestive system and hormone balance.

This is why I recommend both. You want to get nutrients at times without the fiber slowing things down and making the process of nutrient absorption less efficient. But then at other times, you want the fiber for all the benefits it brings!

Difference #2: The Ingredients

Juices give you much more scope to use certain tougher vegetables, like carrot and beets, and the stringier (and therefore impossible to blend) ingredients like celery and wheatgrass.

Smoothies allow you to get arguably more creative with things like nuts, seeds, fats and oils, powders, and supplements. My smoothies regularly contain things like almonds, cashews, chia, cacao, maca, and softer ingredients like avocado.

Generally speaking, you can't blend carrots and celery too well, and too many leafy greens like kale don't work as well in smoothies. And of course, juicing cacao powder, avocado, or chia seeds doesn't really work either.

But all of these ingredients are beneficial. Again, this is why I recommend you enjoy *both* juices and smoothies in your lifestyle.

OTHER EQUIPMENT

First Honorable Mention: the Zoodle Maker

The zoodle maker, or spiralizer, isn't essential, but it is relatively cheap and great to have. To be able to churn out mountains of zucchini noodles or carrot noodles (or any other kind of "oodle") in minutes is fantastic. I use one all the time for salads, curries, and stir-fries. And I almost always use zucchini noodles in place of spaghetti. It gives me natural, gluten-free "pasta," adds an extra serving of nutrient-dense vegetables to my meal, and tastes great.

Alternately, you can use a serrated vegetable peeler to get a similar effect. It is more effort, but you still end up with zoodles.

Second Honorable Mention: the Sprouter!

Sprouts are awesome. And purchasing a sprouter makes growing sprouts incredibly easy. You can grab a simple sprouting jar for under $20 or get an automatic sprouter (which does the watering and misting for you) for between $100 to $200. The fact that this enables you to grow an abundance of sprouts at home with very little effort means it really should be on your shopping list.

THE ESSENTIAL SUPPLEMENTS

I'm sure I'm not alone when I say I have an embarrassing supplement cupboard that could probably fill a walk-in closet. We've all been there. There are so many interesting, intriguing, well-marketed, shiny-looking (and, I'm sure, too-good-to-be-true) supplements out there. And I'm as much a sucker for them as anyone!

However, I want to spare you this affliction of supplement-itis and keep it 20/80. The reality is, if you follow the Alkaline Life Plan for even half the time, you will be getting more than enough of the most important nutrients every day.

As the saying goes, "Supplements are there to supplement, not replace," and there's so much truth to this.

However, I still believe supplements are important and essential for the following reasons:

1. Some nutrients are just *so important* to get on a daily basis, we want to make sure we have a baseline safety net each day.
2. Some nutrients are just *so difficult* to get on a daily basis.
3. Some nutrients can be *incredibly useful* to supplement short term to help you quickly get to a goal.

I've created a more in-depth guide to supplements, including more depth of information on the core supplements and the brands I trust, plus a breakdown of my recommendations for each of the goals we discuss in Part II of this book, at www.alkalinelifebook.com.

The Core Alkaline Life Supplements

Green Powders / Green Drinks

This is the big-boy, most important supplement. I recommend this for everyone. A green drink is a powdered supplement usually made of a combination of grasses, vegetables, fruits, algae, and other foods. The combinations range from just one food (wheatgrass, barley grass, spirulina, etc.) to dozens (some contain over 50 different ingredients). I recommend looking for something in between—about 8 to 10 ingredients is a good sweet spot. That way, you're not spreading the nutrient spectrum per serving too wide or too thin.

With green drinks, it's paramount that you source an organic, non-GMO blend. And while I love to see all different grasses, vegetables, and sprouts in these powders, there are a few ingredients I *don't* love to see in green drinks:

- **High Fruit Content.** A little is okay, but preferably, there isn't any. Low-sugar fruits like tomato, lime, lemon, and grapefruit are fine, but I don't like to see a lot of higher-sugar fruits in there.

- **Mushrooms.** Again, a little medicinal mushroom is fine (reishi, cordyceps, etc.), but this shouldn't be a big component. I also believe medicinal mushrooms should be used in specific bursts for specific goals, not used day in, day out.

- **Algae.** Spirulina and chlorella are acid forming. Yes, they do contain minerals, but those in question are abundant in other greens and grasses.

- **Adaptogens.** You need to be careful with certain herbs and the quantities in which you consume them. Adaptogens such as ashwagandha absolutely need to be cycled (for example, two weeks on, two weeks off). I *highly* recommend you do not consume them daily, long term.

- **Xylitol.** This sweetener is highly refined and not really tested long term for human health. It makes for a good toothpaste but has not been proven yet as a safe sweetener.

The best bet is to keep it quite simple with your greens. The majority of the benefit should come from the grasses, so look to a brand that keeps mostly grass-based.

Alkaline Minerals

The core alkaline minerals are *essential* for fighting inflammation, acidity, and oxidative stress in the body, and I recommend supplementing with these. Look for a product that contains a mix of three or more of the most alkaline-forming minerals: sodium, potassium, magnesium, and calcium.

Alkaline minerals are often a little low in a regular multivitamin product, but they're so important throughout the body, and many of us are deficient in at least one of them. Magnesium and potassium are often lacking in the diet, and a chronic deficiency of them is a marker for inflammatory conditions.[1]

If you can have even just one scoop of an alkaline mineral daily, it will bring a remarkable, noticeable difference to your health, especially with digestive or fatigue conditions.

Omegas and Healthy Fats

Omegas and healthy fats are the next most important to supplement, and the truth is, they're really a food. You can add tons of different sources of these nutrients to your recipes, *but* they are so important that I highly recommend you supplement too.

In terms of omega-3, please try to buy the very best you can afford. You really do get what you pay for. It's best to find a high-quality, tested, researched source if you're buying fish oils, and organic is a must for plant oils. I like to mix up my omega-3 intakes from different sources, but I always include a phospholipid omega-3 each day now too. My daily regimen might look something like:

- 1000 mg flax oil
- 2000 mg omega-3 from fish oil or krill oil
- 500 mg phospholipids

Sometimes, though, I include 1000 mg of phospholipids and less straight omega-3 instead.

The phospholipids are important, as they can more easily cross the blood-brain barrier and carry the oils where they need to go to support cognitive health.

For coconut oil, go organic and make sure it's 100 percent coconut oil or MCT oil (nothing else added).

Tony's Story

I'm currently 62 years young. I started my alkaline journey back in 2005, when my wife was given a short time to live with cancer—six months. I researched, and we started the alkaline way of living.

After many years of yo-yoing with alcohol and alkalizing, we decided to do Ross's alkaline way. My goals were to stop drinking alcohol, drop a few inches on my waist, and get rid of pains in my body.

Seven weeks in, and I've got what I wanted. I'm experiencing zero cravings for anything other than juices and smoothies, my energy is good, I'm sleeping better, and I dropped at least two inches off my waist. I've had so many comments on how healthy I look, and I'm feeling great!

I've tried giving up booze many times over the years since my wife passed, buts it's always been a white-knuckle ride. I've tried everything, but always felt like I was missing out. But for the first time in 15 years, I'm enjoying sobriety, and the cravings have gone. I'm enjoying eating the alkaline foods. Maybe this should part of the 12-step program: Step 13—living alkaline!

What Do Cravings *Really* Mean?

As you move through the 14-Day Alkaline Life Plan, you'll likely notice cravings starting to disappear. Cravings almost *always* mean that your body lacks alkaline minerals such as iron, calcium, magnesium, manganese, potassium, sodium, or zinc.

If you have these cravings, see what they might mean:

Salty food = boron, potassium, and magnesium
Sweet foods = magnesium and zinc
Soda = potassium, magnesium, calcium, and zinc
Cheese and dairy = calcium and iron (particularly important for vegans!)
Dark chocolate = magnesium
Sugar = boron, phosphorus, and zinc
Red meat = iron and zinc (or manganese, if you're stressed)
Fried food = magnesium or iron
Wheat or cereal = phosphorus and iron (and zinc)
Desserts = potassium

Curcumin

Curcumin is the compound within turmeric that has the strongest anti-inflammatory capacity, which is why it's isolated from the whole root for supplementary purposes. When people refer to a curcumin or turmeric supplement, they're effectively saying the same thing.

There have been hundreds of research studies showing the anti-inflammatory power of curcumin, and you just can't go without it while you're fighting inflammation (or want to keep it out).[2, 3, 4]

Alkaline Protein Powders

Alkaline protein powders aren't essential for most, but there also needs to be a little explanation. Your decision to use a protein powder is entirely up to you. It might be because you're hitting the gym or have been advised to consume some after a challenging health condition. Whatever the reason, you can absolutely be alkaline and use protein powders.

The only rules are:

- *No dairy.* Whey is *super* acid forming.
- *No artificial ingredients.* No flavorings, no preservatives, no colors.
- Sprouted and *organic.*

If you follow these rules, you're set. I know the concept of no flavorings is a big one for some, but think of protein powder as what you add to your beautiful-tasting alkaline smoothies rather than something you just mix with water on the run.

The Supporting Cast

I could recommend a million different supplements for a million different reasons (and that's probably why I have the walk-in closet filled with them), but these five are my next most recommended. If the budget permits, they are also smart choices:

- Magnesium (glycinate for all-around use; threonate for sleep and cognitive benefits)
- Vitamin D
- Zinc (ideally, picolinate)
- Selenium
- Psyllium husks

To make your supplement regime more affordable, you can do what I do—take one day per week completely off, and then one week per quarter completely off. I think it's great to give it a break and mix it up to keep your body on its toes!

> For my more detailed guide to supplements, including my recommendations for specific goals and the brands and products I trust, go to www.thealkalinelifebook.com.

· CHAPTER 8 ·

Making It Real
and Your Next Questions

Now you know the fundamentals of what the Alkaline Life are. You understand the science and the logic, and you've read the beautiful stories from some of my beautiful students. You know the most important foods and drinks to aim for and avoid, and you know how to stock your kitchen and the supplements that can support you.

You've seen the big picture of why it's important to avoid an acid-forming lifestyle and provide your body with the nutrients to help support its balancing act.

This is the foundation, and it's fantastic to have this big picture. However, it's also important to have some of the little details. And before we progress to Part II, where we'll dive into the most important health goals and challenges and how the Alkaline Life can help, let's jump into some of the questions that I've heard most frequently starting with a very big and very common one!

HOW LONG DOES IT TAKE TO "GET ALKALINE"?

It depends on how long you've been eating an SMD and living an acid-forming lifestyle, and what impact it's had on you (i.e., are your goals to decrease reflux or weight, or to address something like a hormonal imbalance?). And it depends on what your definition of "get alkaline" is.

Every journey is different, so try not to have specific expectations. For some people, energy jumps quickly once the body is getting these lovely nutrients. For others, energy goes *down* for a while as the body pushes all of its resources toward detoxification and healing.

It really does come down to the individual, what your past health choices were, and of course, how fervently you jump into living alkaline.

In terms of quantifiable, measurable results with your pH, you'll notice some quirks. Most people's urine pH goes *down* before it goes up, which can at first seem disheartening if you don't understand what's going on.

If you have been living an acidic lifestyle for any length of time, you will have built up stored acidic toxins in your body, especially uric acid. As your body recognizes that it is receiving lots of lovely alkaline nutrients, it gets the message that it is now safe to release these toxins, and it does so primarily in the urine. Hence, when you first start to live the Alkaline Life, your urine pH will go *down*. The body looks to expel stored acidity as soon as possible.

However, within a few days, you'll soon notice it starting to track back up again, and before long, you'll be consistently at the target pH for your urine (and saliva if you're testing that too).

HOW DO I TEST MY pH?

The answer is, quite simply: pH testing strips! These are designed to test your saliva and urine (not water*) and are relatively inexpensive.

---

* The pH testing strips work with the enzymes and fluids from your body and do not work with water. To test your drinking water's pH, you can use either a digital meter or testing drops, for which I provide recommendations at www.thealkalinelifebook.com.

However, there's a right and a wrong way to use them. I get messages practically daily from people confused about their pH, because they're using these strips incorrectly. Now, I don't mean that they're peeing on them wrong! But they are using them at the wrong time and under the wrong conditions.

The urine test is a decent measure of alkalinity and progress with your diet, and I prefer this over using a saliva test. In a nutshell, your urine pH reading is an indicator of your progress from being stuck in diet-induced acidity and living in the "safe" zone to your progression out of the safe zone and up to that perfect pH of 7.365 to 7.4. When you're eating an acid-forming diet and living in the safe zone of DIA, your body will expel a lot of acidity through the urine. When the body starts the process of eliminating stored toxins and acidity, your urine will also show as acidic.

So, while you're in those two states, your urine pH will be below where you want it. You want your urine pH to be around pH 7.2 to pH 7.6.[1] If you are getting regular urine pH readings around this level, you know you're on the right track.

However, as with any scientific test, it is essential to stay in control of your variables. You want to test your urine under the same conditions each day. I believe the most important urine reading is your first of the day, as it truly demonstrates the acidity (or not) that your body has expelled overnight. So it is a good idea to test each time with your first urine of the day.

Saliva pH can be useful in some settings, but it is largely inconsistent and less relevant than urine pH readings. Saliva pH really is more of a measure of what you have consumed in the past half hour or so.

Getting the wrong, or misleading, information is worse than no information at all. If you're trying to get alkaline and are making mistakes, but your tests are inaccurately showing you're getting more alkaline, then you'll keep on making those same mistakes forever. Or worse, you'll step it up a notch and do more of what is not working and end up going even faster in the wrong direction.

And I can assure you, people get this test wrong all the time.

Just today I spoke to a client who was rinsing their mouth with water before testing.

Sounds good, right? Nope. This would at best give her the instant reaction of her salivary gland to the tap water, and at worst (and most likely) simply a read of the tap water itself.

Alongside the quality of your test by keeping the variables stable, you also need to consider the frequency of testing. So many people excitedly get their pH testing strips and start testing themselves every five minutes.

This is not helpful. You want to test yourself consistently and look for the long-term trend. Measure yourself consistently (for example, each morning or every other morning) for a month, and see how you change over time. You should neither get too excited or too stressed about each individual result; you just want to see that gradual improvement over time.

> I've created an in-depth guide to pH testing for you, which you can download for free at www.thealkalinelifebook.com.

HOW DO I MEASURE 20/80 IN MY DIET?

My Alkaline Life Club members must have asked how to measure 20/80 in a thousand different ways, but the most common question by far is, "If I have a coffee, can I eat something alkaline after it to make it okay?"

I love the thought process, and there is some logic to it. But the thing is, the body doesn't react in the moment to every little thing we eat. Yes, there is a digestive reaction (as you'll discover shortly), and yes, there is the acidity produced by metabolizing some of these foods. But the more important things are the longer-term, overall picture of your diet and the volume of acid-forming to alkaline-forming foods and drinks you consume.

In short, try not to think in the immediate short term; look at the bigger picture. We don't want to fall into the trap of micro-analyzing every single ingredient in every single meal. We would never have a treat or any flexibility if we did that. We want to see it as an overall, "Today, did I eat *mostly* alkaline-forming foods?"

You certainly can apply the 20/80 by making sure each plate is 80 percent alkaline-forming foods. For some people, this is a help. But the reality is, you don't need to be as specific as this. You will still get incredible results if you just commit to having *mostly* alkaline-forming foods and drinks and keeping the acid-forming foods to a minimum.

CAN YOU GET TOO ALKALINE? ARE THERE ANY SIDE EFFECTS?

It is physically possible to get too alkaline. This condition is called—surprise, surprise—*diet-induced alkalosis*. However, it's very rare and practically impossible. You would need to be making incredibly unusual dietary choices to force this to happen. For most people, even if they tried to do it, they would still fail.

There are two reasons why. First, the body has far more easily accessible buffers to reduce pH than it does to raise pH. If you eat a huge number of alkaline foods, your body, if it had to, would very easily adjust the pH back down without breaking a sweat, because we always have acidity at hand to do this job. The body creates a lot of acidity by design, through our natural daily bodily functions.

Second, when you look at the pH of the most *alkaline* foods, you'll find they're all only mildly alkaline forming. If you're eating kale and spinach, avocado, and cucumber, these are all very mildly alkaline (pH 7.2 to pH 8.0). This is only a little over neutral and is gently supporting your alkaline balance.

Compare this with typical acid-forming foods and drinks such as coffee and cola, sugar, and sweets, which are between pH 3 and pH 4. Remember on page 20 where we discussed the pH scale being logarithmic? This means pH 6 is 10 times more acidic than neutral, pH 5 is 100 times, pH 4 is 1,000 times, and pH 3 is 10,000 times more acidic. Natural alkaline foods are gently supporting your body's pH buffering, while the modern, processed foods are all incredibly acidic.

Consider that the body *can* buffer blood pH back up to a safe level, even when we eat foods that are 10,000 times more acidic than it would like. So it stands to reason that the buffering in the case of overalkalizing is not a problem. Even if you somehow managed to get to alkalosis (again, practically impossible with food), it would be the equivalent of your body doing the work that a couple of sips of soda would require.

In other words, don't worry about being *too alkaline*.

THE BIG PICTURE BEFORE WE GET STARTED

Before we jump into Part II, where we'll deep-dive into 10 of the most common health challenges and how we apply the Alkaline Life to them, I want to come back to the core foundations. These are the fundamentals of the Alkaline Life.

So far, we've looked at what the Alkaline Life is and what diet-induced acidosis is.

We've looked at the practical applications of living alkaline, and diet-induced acidosis and the science, data, and studies.

We've seen a few of my students' stories and how powerful living alkaline can be.

Now Is the Time to Start Applying the 80/20 of the Alkaline Life!

I have given you a fair amount of detail, data, studies, and the biology about how the alkaline balance works in the body. You don't need to try to remember everything. Just remember the big picture!

If you eat purely natural foods, you will be avoiding 80 percent of the foods on the acid-forming list. We are not adding sugar, gluten, chemicals, preservatives, nitrates, processed fats, flavorings, colorings, and so on to meals we make ourselves at home.

Even if you totally ignore everything else here and simply cook everything you eat from scratch, you'll get it right almost all the time. Let's sum it up.

Add more:

- *Leafy greens*: kale, spinach, arugula, lettuce, watercress, chard; any other greens
- *Cruciferous veggies*: broccoli and broccoli sprouts, cauliflower, cabbage, Brussels sprouts, bok choy
- *Low-sugar fruits*: avocado, lemons, and limes; berries such as blueberries and strawberries
- *Anti-inflammatory foods*: turmeric, ginger, asparagus, garlic
- *Antioxidant-rich foods*: bell pepper, carrots, kale, tomatoes
- *Healthy fats*: omega-3 from leafy greens, nuts, seeds, oily fish; saturated fats from coconut

In short—lots of fresh veggies; natural, whole, plant-based foods; plenty of high-water-content foods; and lots of healthy fats.

Eat less:

- Processed foods
- Packaged foods
- Sugar
- Gluten
- Refined and processed fats
- Meat and dairy

We Tend to Overcomplicate

As humans, we tend to overvalue complexity and undervalue simplicity. We often assume that something that is more complex must be better or more valuable than something simple.

Please try to fight this "complexity bias." You certainly *can* make living alkaline as complex as you like. You could implement it to the nth degree, calculating all of the food pH, measuring weight to make sure you get the right percentage of acid to alkaline. You could implement an elaborate routine and test your saliva and urine pH several times a day.

You could.

But you absolutely do not need to. I have worked with enough people over the past two decades to say, with absolute certainty, that you will get the same result by applying the 80/20 (or, as we call it, the 20/80) approach.

In Part II, we deep-dive into the most common goals my students in the Alkaline Life Club come to me with. And after we've done the deep dive into *your* goal, we'll get into action.

It's incredibly exciting, so let's take the leap.

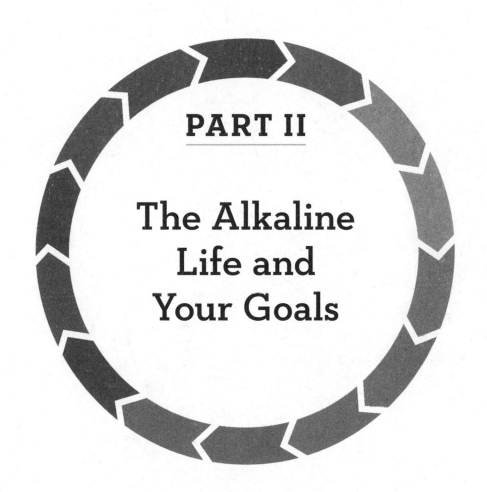

PART II

The Alkaline
Life and
Your Goals

· CHAPTER 9 ·

We Have the Power!

Now that we understand the fundamentals of the Alkaline Life, let's explore how they apply to some of the most common health challenges that people face. Each of these challenges is unique but shares the same foundations of imbalance in the body: inflammation, oxidative stress, and diet-induced acidosis.

I want you to feel confident we can make a huge impact on your health through diet and living the Alkaline Life. So many of my clients have been told, "There's nothing you can do"—and that they must simply live with medication and pain. We often hear that a condition can't be cured or that it's genetic. And while there is, of course, some truth to these in many instances, I believe they are overstated.

What I am sure of is that through our diet and how we live, we can reduce or remove the symptoms. You can create a situation where you live each day as if the condition doesn't exist. It may still be there somewhere, lurking in the background, but you may be able to get to a point of living with minimal symptoms. And for me, that is a great result.

I should point out, once again, that you should always follow the advice of your doctor, physician, or consultant. But you should also never accept the concept that you cannot, at the very least, *support* your body with nutrition. Eating and living in the best way possible will support your body, no matter your treatment plan.

ABUNDANT HEALTH IS IN YOUR HANDS

By far the biggest health challenges we face are:

- Atherosclerotic disease (cardiovascular disease and cerebrovascular disease)
- Cancer
- Neurodegenerative disease (Alzheimer's disease being the most common)

As a society, we tend to see these diseases as fate. If we're diagnosed with one, it's bad luck, inevitable, and there's nothing we can do. It's genetics, and that's all there is to it. Right?

If you look back as far as you can in the record at the members of your family tree who have sadly died, you will see trends—if there's a predisposition to cancer or heart disease, and so on. And genetics can certainly play a role. I heard a saying that "genetics may load the gun, but they don't pull the trigger," and while this may be giving genetics more credit than perhaps it deserves, *yes*, we do have some genetic predispositions.

But that does not tell the whole story. It does not take into account that *diet and lifestyle are the biggest variables.*

If we look at our biggest health challenges, consider these statistics of how preventable they are through diet:

Cancer: up to 95 percent[1]
Type 2 diabetes: 90 percent[2]
Heart disease: 82 percent[3]
Stroke: 80 percent (or more)[4]
Alzheimer's disease: up to 99 percent[5]

We should live in power, not fear. And remember, while biology, diseases, and your body are all incredibly complex, the solutions are simple. If we reduce and remove diet-induced acidity, chronic inflammation, and oxidative stress, your body will be in a position of power, strength, and vitality, and your health risks will drop significantly.

LIVING ALKALINE MEANS LIVING YOUNGER

We all want to stay young. We all want to prevent aging and turn back the clock. But what does that really mean? When I teach my students in the Alkaline Life Club, we think about what our goals really are. It isn't just to lose weight or to beat a challenge like irritable bowel syndrome (IBS) or fibromyalgia.

The goal is to feel good, to have energy—to feel strong, fit, and vital, to have mental clarity and cognitive health, and to live life at its fullest for as long as we can.

As you read through the case studies in this book, you'll see amazing health transformations of beating cancer, heart disease, autoimmune disease, osteoporosis, brain tumors, pain, and arthritis. But it's the bit behind the result that I love—people being able to follow their passions, spend time playing with their grandkids, have freedom to move and exercise, and relish being in nature. The impact on their quality of life is so inspiring and motivational, it gets me to keep on getting better at what I do!

So, again, the concept of reversing aging and increasing life span isn't just about living longer. It's about living better, with more zest, vitality, and vigor. On the whole, 80 percent of our health and quality of life in the last 20 years of our lives has been due to our lifestyle and the choices we've made. Less than 20 percent has been genetic. It is well and truly in our hands.

How We Look

While it might seem a little based in ego, our physical appearance is a relevant and worthy marker for a lot of people, particularly when it is about how we look at ourselves rather than how others see us. We can assume that others think we look great (or not; that's up to them), but how we look and feel within our own skin is important, and as you've seen already, so much research points to alkaline-forming foods and drinks as having a wonderfully positive impact on skin elasticity, preventing or even slowing gray hair, fine lines and wrinkles, skin tone and color, hair and nail strength, and cellulite appearance.

Bone Strength

Possibly the first main area of funded study into the alkaline diet was around the link to bone strength, and subsequent high-quality studies have been published verifying this.[6, 7, 8, 9]

But it goes beyond that, because having weaker bones is exponentially detrimental to both length of life and quality. Hip fracture after 65 years increases risk of death in the next 12 months to between 40 and 60 percent.[10] But it also, of course, has a significant impact on quality of life. Remember, we don't just want to live a long time; we want the time to be of the highest quality too.

Muscle Mass

While it's slightly more strongly correlated with men than women, a loss of muscle mass as we age is also associated with an increased risk of all-cause mortality. And again, think about the things that make us feel older. A loss of strength is certainly one of them. Living alkaline has long been proven to preserve muscle mass in older men and women[11, 12] and help promote muscle growth in younger ones too![13]

As a little bonus, as a study published in the *Journal of Sports Science and Medicine* showed that living alkaline also promotes athletic performance.[14] The researchers had subjects live alkaline for a nine-day period and assessed their athletic performance before and after. They found that the alkaline diet increased anaerobic exercise performance and resulted in a lower respiratory exchange ratio (RER), which means the body turns to fat for fuel instead of carbohydrate (which is what you really, really want). A little pleasure I got from this study was that the authors wrote that the results were "contrary to their expectation."

There are many other studies showing the alkaline way speeding recovery times and increasing aerobic performance.[15, 16, 17] But I love this study for highlighting the RER impact, because burning fat for fuel is so critically important.

Cognitive Health

Of course, if we're constantly tired and forgetful, have foggy thinking, and are losing that mental sharpness, we'll feel like we're aging. More importantly, cognitive decline and neurodegenerative disease will certainly speed that feeling of aging. As we'll get to further in Part II, the alkaline diet is strongly correlated with a protection against neurodegenerative diseases such as Alzheimer's, Parkinson's, and more.

Aches and Pains

In psychological studies around what makes people feel older, experiencing pain, aches, and a loss of physical vitality always top the list. If we're creaking out of bed, feeling back pain and stiff joints, and having constant, niggling injuries, we will feel old.

When we look at longevity as both length of life (life span) and quality of life (health span), and we check the five boxes of keeping up our skin and appearance, bone strength, muscle mass, cognitive health, and aches and pains, we will feel considerably younger—emotionally and physically. Our health span is increased, and we feel better. And if we can lower the risk of, help prevent, and even reverse the most common and serious degenerative and foundational diseases, we will extend our life span.

So as we get into the most common, debilitating, and challenging health conditions and how they can be supported by the Alkaline Life, remember that the goal here is not only to extend your life span but also to increase the quality of your life.

Over the next 10 chapters, I walk you through the 10 most common goals my Alkaline Life Club members come to me for support with. I demonstrate the role of diet-induced acidosis and dive into the specifics for addressing each goal and the nutrients to focus on with the Alkaline Life Plan.

Of course you can skip around to the chapters specific to your health challenge or goal, but I really recommend that you read through them all, as there is plenty to learn by looking at each of these conditions and their relationship to diet-induced acidosis. And you might be able to identify a condition or goal that you hadn't thought of before!

IMPORTANT: THE 20/80 ACTIONS BOX

Before we start digging into each of the goals and challenges, I want to draw your attention to the 20/80 Actions box at the end of every chapter. The all-encompassing Alkaline Life Plan in Part III is the foundational plan for every goal, symptom, and challenge. Because as we've discovered, no matter the challenge, DIA often plays a role, and an alkaline life can help to be the solution.

However, we can speed our results, and focus on our specific goal too, by taking specific actions and including specific nutrients.

This is what the 20/80 Actions are. They are the handful of 20/80 steps that I recommend for particular goals. They are the needle-movers, the big dominos that will give you way more bang for your buck. So, whichever your primary goal is, you can add these 20/80 Actions on top of the Alkaline Life Plan steps as much as you see fit. Think of them as little boosters to your progress.

And this often raises the question, "Which goal should I go for first?" It truly does not matter. Don't let that be a source of procrastination or let yourself get bogged down in the detail. You can keep it really simple and *just* do the Alkaline Life Plan steps, and once you feel comfortable, start adding in some more of the specifics from our little 20/80 boxes later in the process.

Whichever goal you go for, with the Alkaline Life Plan, you'll make progress across the board. As the saying goes, a rising tide lifts all ships.

· CHAPTER 10 ·

Excess Weight and Obesity

Over two billion people worldwide are now overweight, and the number is growing each year. In the U.S. alone, there are concurrently over a hundred million people "dieting" at any given time. But things are not improving; they're actually getting worse.

It's time to accept that the way we've been doing things is *not* working.

Excess weight is a symptom of imbalance.

Read that again.

It is not a result of eating too much fat or too many calories, or anything else. It is a symptom of imbalance.

When we're in a state of chronic, metabolic diet-induced acidosis, there are so many factors that can lead our body to create and stubbornly retain fat cells, and they all have acidosis at their root.

The weight gain could come from thyroid imbalance, digestive issues, inflammation, oxidative stress, autoimmune conditions, adrenal fatigue, or a combination of three or four of these.

And then, even more frustratingly, in a state of diet-induced acidosis, the conditions are such that it becomes practically impossible to shift the weight—your body clings on to fat cells for dear life.

It is *incredibly* frustrating. That is, until you restore your alkaline balance.*

The fact remains that "calories in, calories out" (CICO) is too often oversimplified. While there's obvious mechanical truth to the fact that if you burn more calories than you consume, you'll lose weight, this doesn't mean that the weight loss will be a loss of fat—or that it will be sustained.

Calorie-restrictive dieting simply does not work. The data tells us that in over 99 percent of cases, when people lose weight through calorie-restrictive dieting, they regain all of the weight, or more, within 18 months.[1]

YOUR BODY'S POINT OF VIEW

For us to lose unwanted body fat and maintain our ideal weight for the long term, we need to start with the most important question: *Why* has the body created fat cells and held on to them? When we understand *why* the body does this, we can start to see how to give the body what it needs to release this fat.

Again, it's all about working with what the body needs to return to balance and thrive.

When we look at it from this perspective (what the body *needs*), fat loss becomes simple.

There are many ways that diet-induced acidosis leads to fat gain and retention, and if you want or need to lose weight, you have a combination of these factors that is unique to you. For some people the root cause of the fat gain is just one factor, and for others, it's a multitude.

Let's look at a few of the ways in which DIA causes excess weight.

---

* It's important to point out here that the Alkaline Life is not a weight-loss program. It's a body-balancing program. If you have weight to lose, you absolutely can lose it, quickly and sustainably. But being underweight is as much of a symptom of imbalance as being overweight. If you are underweight, you won't lose more weight by living alkaline; the opposite will happen. For both over- and underweight individuals, the Alkaline Life will help return you to your natural, thriving weight.

Adrenal Fatigue

When it comes to excess weight, the effect of DIA on your endocrine system is rapid and devastating. Calories in versus calories out achieves absolutely nothing if adrenal fatigue is the underlying cause of the weight gain and retention.

As we mentioned earlier, when our body is in a state of acidosis, this signals the adrenals to produce excess cortisol. Chronically elevated cortisol puts incredible stress on the adrenals. It's effectively your body in fight-or-flight mode all day, all night, and nonstop.

When we're in fight-or-flight mode, the body clings on to fat for dear life and will not let go of it. If you do manage to lose any weight, your body will scurry to put it back on as quickly as possible. The message is that famine is coming, there's danger ahead, and you need to preserve yourself.

When we start to live by the principles of the Alkaline Life and support the body's pH balance, cortisol stops being produced, the adrenals have the space and time to repair, we come out of fight or flight, and the fat can be released.

Weight-Loss Hormone Disruption

If you want to lose weight, you need to know about two essential hormones: leptin and ghrelin. These are affectionately known as the hunger hormones or weight-loss hormones, and they're fascinating.

Ghrelin is the true hunger hormone. It signals to your brain that you're hungry and need to eat. Too much ghrelin, and you'll eat more than you need.

Leptin is the satiety hormone or starvation hormone. It tells your brain you are full and don't need to eat any more. Too little leptin, and you'll never feel full.

You can see where I'm heading here. An acidic, inflammatory, standard modern diet of gluten, sugar, processed foods, toxins, and so on leads to that situation of too much ghrelin and not enough leptin.

That makes it a little tricky to lose weight. Can you imagine trying to eat healthily but you're always hungry, and when you eat, you never feel full?

If you feel like you're always struggling with cravings and have no willpower, this is just another of the times I want you to know that it isn't your fault.

The Gut-Brain Connection and Your Weight

The gut and brain are connected to such a degree that many consider them to be the same organ. They communicate via a two-way street called the "gut-brain axis" and influence mood, health, and cognition through a dance of neurotransmitters, hormones, and microbes.

When it comes to your weight, ghrelin is a good example of the gut-brain connection. Only discovered in 1999, it's made in the gut and stimulates responses in the brain's pituitary gland and hypothalamus. Again, the more ghrelin you have in your system, the hungrier you are. It is supposed to rise before meals and drop after them, but when it is disrupted by acidosis, the drop doesn't occur. So if you find yourself fighting cravings and can't seem to stay away from the fridge after dinner, it's probably due to elevated ghrelin levels.

Leptin is also a recent discovery; it was found in 1994. For quite some time, it was a confusing hormone. Leptin is produced in adipose tissue (fat), and the more fat a person has, the more leptin they produce. But hang on—don't we *want* to have more leptin, so we feel full?

You can imagine that when a hormone was discovered that makes us feel full, Big Pharma companies were in a space race to produce leptin-in-a-bottle. Alas, their excitement was short-lived, as soon after, leptin resistance was discovered.[2] Fat actually blocks the signal of leptin, so the more fat cells you have, the more leptin resistant you become. And with leptin resistance, your brain gets no leptin signaling. It thinks you're always hungry, and you're driven to eat—all the time.

Adiponectin is also worth mentioning here. It's also produced in adipose tissue, but in those who are overweight or obese, its levels are very low. Adiponectin is responsible for regulating insulin sensitivity, lipid metabolism, and other weight-related tasks—and it is also responsible for telling the body to burn fat for fuel! With low adiponectin, the body becomes far less effective at utilizing and burning fat. But as we heal, rebalance, and support the body, it begins to access adiponectin again and can burn your excess fat cells for fuel.

Shouldn't We Just Cut Calories?

The "solution" to losing weight for many decades has been to eat fewer calories than you burn. While mechanically this works for a while, it's flawed as a sustainable weight-loss solution.

Here are a few myths I will quickly debunk to help you stop worrying about—and counting—calories:

Myth #1: Excess calories are always fundamentally used up by the creation of fat cells.

The standard calorie-deficit diet approach to weight loss assumes that any calories over your arbitrary, static basal metabolic rate[3] are automatically used by the body to create fat cells. Consume over 2,000 calories, and it automatically becomes fat, right?

But why would the body do this? A calorie is simply a measure of energy potential in the body and this energy can be used to regulate hundreds of processes including bone production, heat production, digestion, metabolism, protein synthesis, liver and kidney detoxification, breathing, and cognition.

To assume that whenever there's an excess of energy, it's used solely to produce fat cells rather than to undertake any of the other hundreds of processes the body uses energy for is bizarre.

If we eat the volume of food that gives us 500 extra calories today, who is to determine whether that extra energy is used to create bowel movements, process the additional protein that might be in those calories, or turned into fat cells?

Myth #2: Calories in and calories out operate independently.

If you lower calories in, the calories out will stay stable and you'll lose weight, right? Alas, not so much. When you lower your calories *in*, your body regulates your calories *out* downward to match it. This process can take a week or two, but it gets there.[4] This is why calorie-deficit diets only work for a couple of weeks.

Myth #3: Restricting calories gives sustainable weight loss.

We all know intuitively that when we crash diet by dramatically decreasing calories, it isn't a long-term solution. So why would we try to lose weight for the long term by lowering calories—or focusing on calories at all? Not only is it unsustainable to keep up, but scientifically, the studies also show that it programs our body to *regain* all of the lost weight!

After a period of caloric restriction, the body's levels of several hormones associated with satiety, appetite, insulin, blood sugar, and more, including leptin, peptide YY, cholecystokinin, insulin, ghrelin, gastric inhibitory polypeptide, and pancreatic polypeptide, have been found to head in all the wrong directions.[5, 6]

In other words, due to calorie restriction, you can become practically hardwired to regain weight instead of losing it.

Myth #4: A calorie is a calorie.

So many weight-loss diets are based on pure calorie intake—whether you get those calories from chocolate bars or spinach is irrelevant.

This is so strange.

Remember, a calorie is simply a measure of a unit of energy. So of course, calories gained from a straight sugar drink have a different effect on the body compared to calories gained from a carrot or an apple. This highlights the flawed thinking behind calorie counting more than anything else. Clearly, what's important is the nutritional components of the food you eat and its ability to either heal and bring balance or to create acidity, inflammation, oxidative stress, and imbalance. It isn't the calories; it's what the food does inside your body. Please let go of any thoughts around calorie counting and trust in the Alkaline Life to bring your body back into balance!

Excess Acidity

As mentioned in Chapter 2, the body has a natural acid-buffering system, and we know that it's quickly overwhelmed. Built for the acidity produced by our bodily functions, it can't deal with the standard modern diet. When excess acidity and its toxic by-products cannot be eliminated, the body tries to protect your vital organs by storing the excess and toxicity away in fat cells. Initially it does so in subcutaneous fat (which is safe), but if that becomes overwhelmed, it begins to store it in visceral fat cells, which surround your vital organs. Fatty liver is the first sign that this is occurring.

The good news is that the situation can be quickly addressed. The body is a detoxification machine, and when we start to address the acidosis by giving the body the alkaline nutrients and nourishment it needs, it sends the signal to remove the toxins, and the fat cells go with it!

However, this can begin a vicious cycle.

Chronic Inflammation

We have talked about inflammation a lot already, and we know that a standard modern diet is highly inflammatory. Regardless of your goals, symptoms, or health conditions, we must address inflammation. And the same goes for excess weight.

Inflammation causes the body to create fat cells, and then each of them creates more inflammation . . . *which equals more fat cells*. We must break this loop.

Thanks to inflammatory compounds that get in the way of how insulin works, inflammation in the body can trigger insulin resistance. This results in higher glucose levels and fat accumulation in the liver, both of which contribute to producing even more insulin resistance. This too creates a vicious cycle: as weight gain increases, it fosters more insulin resistance, while insulin resistance leads to increased weight gain.

THE SOLUTION IS THE SAME

When you provide your body with the delicious alkaline nourishment that removes the pressure and stress of fighting acidosis while giving it the tools to heal and rebalance, magic really does happen.

This isn't about calories. Stop thinking and stressing about calories and start thinking about nourishment. When your hormones are balanced, your digestive system soothed, your cortisol levels normalized, your liver operating healthily, and everything back in balance, there is no reason left for your body to create excess fat cells and store them.

When we give the body what it needs to thrive, everything falls into place.

Darline's Story

I live in the middle of a cedar forest where for over 30 years, my husband and I took care of abandoned and injured animals. I lost my husband about 18 months ago, and I was afraid I would have to move and leave the beautiful forest where I live.

In the first year of working with Ross and living his alkaline life, I lost a total of 101 pounds (46 kg) and went from a size 22 to a size 12. In the next year, I lost a further 26 pounds (12 kg), and I am gaining strength I was afraid I would never have again.

Because of the significant reduction in inflammation, I have also significantly reduced my pain level. I can now walk 90 to 95 percent of the time without a walker. My blood pressure and cholesterol levels are now normal, and my liver tests are showing so much improvement.

In the beginning I was worried that there would be so many new things to learn, and it was scary, but the support to take baby steps and the clear, step-by-step guidelines with all of the tools make it possible.

I am 75 years old, and thanks to the Alkaline Life, I am getting my life back.

20/80 ACTIONS FOR EXCESS WEIGHT

Action One: Support Your Adrenals

A daily green juice is ultimately part of the Alkaline Life Plan, and I would love you to incorporate this as soon as you realistically can, especially if weight loss is one of your goals. Your adrenals will *love* you for it, and if you're struggling to lose weight, they definitely need some love. When you consider the nutrients that the adrenals need to repair and rebalance, they are all in abundance in leafy greens, cruciferous plants, and other fruits and vegetables such as cucumbers, bell peppers, carrots, beets, and those potent anti-inflammatories, turmeric and ginger.

You're looking to get lots of lovely alkaline minerals such as zinc, magnesium, potassium, and sodium, and green juice gives you all of those.

Your adrenals are also among the organs with the highest concentration of vitamin C in the body, and they need it to try to maintain balance. Of course, there's a ton of vitamin C in many of the most alkaline foods, but I also recommend using a high-quality vitamin C supplement.

Action Two: Early-A.M. Nourishment

This involves eating within an hour of rising to get your metabolism firing; including at least 20 grams of protein (to help balance cortisol and insulin), healthy fats and fiber, and as many vegetables as possible to encourage pH balance, soothe inflammation, and get the oxidative stress out! Getting these nutrients in early in the morning starts a cascade of benefits that lasts all day and supports your weight loss.

Action Three: Ramp Up Your Metabolism

Ensuring you get essential fats each day is a big part of all this: taking 3 grams of omega-3 and 1 gram of coconut oil daily, plus your naturally consumed fats in avocados, leafy greens, etc. is a huge step in the right direction. These fats also support your adrenals.

Consuming extra leafy greens is a smart choice too, as they contain chlorophyll, magnesium, and iron, which are essential in regulating metabolism.

Action Four: Support the Weight-Loss Hormones

Balancing leptin and ghrelin is so important in the weight-loss journey. Simple steps to do this include proper hydration (dehydration impairs leptin function) and adding anti-inflammatories like turmeric and ginger (as inflammation impairs fat cell function, and leptin signaling to the brain comes from your fat cells) as well as zinc (which is known to support both hormones).

· CHAPTER 11 ·

Fighting Chronic Fatigue

When you've been living in a state of DIA, fatigue is not just probable; it's inevitable. But you can fix it easily, and results can flow quickly. It's not to say a chronic condition like fibromyalgia can be switched off overnight, but you can experience improvement rapidly. I am incredibly confident about addressing fatigue, because I've seen it completely disappear in my clients, and this was the first challenge I healed in my own body when I started to live alkaline almost 20 years ago.

I used to wake up in the morning, and the first thought I had was to count how many hours until I could get back to bed. Not good. And boy, that seems even worse put on paper! But I began fueling my body with the nutrients it needed with small baby steps. First, I fixed my hydration, starting with replacing one or two of my daily coffees (I was having six to eight a day) with rooibos tea. Within a day or two of this, I noticed my usual afternoon energy slump easing.

Then I started adding green juices in the morning. This was all I did for a while, and the impact was profound. Within a few days, my mornings were supercharged. My green juice was the ultimate energy drink.

Inspired by this, I started taking salads to work instead of getting canteen food (sandwiches, chocolate bars, chips, and the like). Then I invested in supplements, getting more healthy fats, drinking green drinks (the powdered supplements I mentioned in Chapter 7), and an antioxidant capsule. Adding the healthy fats helped to stretch out the blood-sugar peaks and troughs I was experiencing and stopped me seeking sugar for energy.

As I noticed my energy improve, it only added to my momentum and confidence, and I had the energy to start exercising and cooking a proper meal after work instead of slumping on the sofa with a takeout or microwave meal.

And as I started to add more and more alkaline meals, slowly replacing the acid-forming foods I'd been living on, my mental clarity returned, my sleep improved, and my fatigue eventually disappeared.

I didn't realize it at the time, but I was focusing on my 20/80 actions and knocking down the big dominos, which made all the next steps so much easier.

You can do the same, and I can't wait to show you how.

WHERE DOES ENERGY COME FROM?

Energy can come from several sources in the body, broadly categorized into:

- Converting energy from the food we consume (glycolysis, the Krebs cycle, and the electron transport chain)
- Converting energy sources stored within the body (amino acids, glycerol, glycogen, fat, lactate, ketones, etc.)

The food (fuel) we give our body has a huge influence on the levels of energy we experience. And then there is a second influence: *how our body uses that energy.*

Barbara's Story

The first time I did the coaching, I was going through a rheumatoid arthritis flare-up. For weeks and months, I could hardly move due to the pain and exhaustion from chronic fatigue syndrome, plus IBS symptoms.

On the 10th day of living alkaline, I woke, and to my surprise, I had hardly any pain. I could move. I checked my body and was amazed that the inflammation and pain had subsided. I actually got up and showered, got dressed, and took my little dog for a gentle walk. For so long I had not been able to go up or down stairs without a rest and lie-down!

The great thing is, these benefits continue. In the years of keeping to alkaline methods, I have not relapsed to using my wheelchair. I can still have the occasional relapse and flare-ups, but these are less severe and soon calmed. My fingers that were clawing have straightened out.

I am a psychologist counselor and work from a positive psychology and CBT [cognitive behavioral therapy] perspective. I am very aware of the benefits of the mind-body connection mainly in family therapy, and with children and young people. I still have mobility in my wrists and hands, spine, and lower body to carry on working and running art therapy workshops!

CAUSES OF FATIGUE IN DIET-INDUCED ACIDOSIS

When we are in a state of acidosis, a huge amount of the energy produced in the body is spent simply trying to survive and operate in this state of imbalance. The additional workload of being in diet-induced acidosis is significant, and so even if you have lots of energy to use, it's all being spent simply trying to rebalance and keep you alive!

The Four Types of Acidosis-Induced Fatigue

In my 20-plus years of coaching, beating fatigue or a desire for more energy is a goal for practically every one of my students.

When we dig into their diet, challenges, history, and goals, the source of their fatigue becomes clear. In almost every single case, it's rooted in one, or a combination, of the following four areas.

Malnourishment Fatigue

Your body needs nutrients to thrive and create energy. Without nutrients, there is none. The most direct way that *malnourishment fatigue* occurs is when we simply do not eat enough nutrients. The body can extract energy from a drive-through burger, but it is incredibly limited (and then the gluten, sugar, preservatives, and additives will rob more energy than they give). But the energy your body gets from a nutrient-dense, alkaline-forming meal is greater and far easier to access.

Simply consuming more nutrients will have a significant impact. However, there is a "but." The body also needs to be able to *extract* the nutrients from the foods we consume. A long-term SMD almost inevitably leads to clogging in the small intestine, and this is not good news.

The small intestine is the part of your digestive system where the nutrient extraction and absorption occurs. Its walls are lined with lots of tiny, finger-like protrusions called *microvilli.*

These are responsible for extracting and absorbing the nutrients from the food we eat, and they expand the surface area of the small intestine dramatically.

When we consume an acid-forming diet, food does not get properly broken down and prepared for this stage of digestion, and the improperly broken-down food gets clogged in the small intestine and flattens the microvilli. This greatly diminishes the capacity of the small intestine to absorb nutrients, meaning that even if you eat all of these nutrient-dense, alkaline-forming foods, only a small percentage of the goodness can be absorbed and used by the body.

Without nutrients, energy conversion is incredibly low, and fatigue sets in.

What makes matters worse is that most acid-forming foods that the SMD relies on (pasta, cereals, breads, etc.) all contain gluten. When gluten is broken down by transglutaminase into its two proteins (glutenin and gliadin), the gut identifies gliadin as dangerous and produces antibodies to attack it. These antibodies then degrade the microvilli and flatten them.[1]

And then there's a further problem: zonulin. As discussed earlier, this is not an outcome we want. Remember, zonulin causes the tight junctures of the small intestine to become degraded (in other words, leaky gut), allowing undigested food and toxins back into the bloodstream, causing an immune response and dramatically increased inflammation. This damage to the junctures compromises the absorption capability of the microvilli further, creating an environment of fatigue, immune overstimulation, and inflammation.

But as you start to heal and repair the gut, the clogged-up junk in your small intestine is broken down and removed, and the tears and gaps in the wall of the small intestine heal and close. Once you are getting the benefits of the nutrients you consume, your energy will skyrocket.

> **Note:** If you're experiencing fatigue or digestive imbalance, I recommend focusing on juices more than smoothies. If you have a clogged-up small intestine situation, the fiber-free nutrients of the juice are far more easily utilized by the body. As the energy starts to return, you can add more smoothies in too.

Mental Fatigue

When we think of tiredness and fatigue, a lot of it is related to how we feel mentally. *Mental fatigue* affects all of us from time to time, of course. But it shouldn't be a daily occurrence. Sadly, for many people, it is.

Mental fatigue occurs when the brain is underpowered and the body is constantly exposed to foods, drinks, and chemicals that rob the body of the fuels that the mitochondria need to power up our adenosine triphosphate (ATP).

In a nutshell, mitochondria are *organelles*. These tiny structures are present in practically every cell in the body and provide them with the things they need. One of their key roles is to generate ATP from the foods we consume. ATP is the carrier of the energy created to fuel our body. ATP is crucial to energy, and when the mitochondria are negatively impacted, this significantly impacts their capacity to produce ATP. Thus our energy plummets, especially the energy needed by the brain.[2]

It's important to note that our food choices are by far the most significant influence on our mitochondria. If you're not producing ATP, it's because of what you're eating. Giving the body the conditions in which the mitochondria thrive and ATP can be effortlessly produced, and then effortlessly get to work, is key to experiencing energy and vitality.

Consuming an acid-forming diet is literally the opposite of what the mitochondria want. A state of DIA is devastating to the body's mitochondria factory. What was previously an assumption has now been proven in several very well-received studies.[3, 4, 5]

When we look at some of the common additives in packaged, processed foods, it's hardly surprising. Inorganic phosphates (which are very different from the phosphates found naturally in food) are added to up to 80 percent of packaged foods as a preservative and stabilizer, and when consumed in large amounts, they cause severe mitochondrial damage.[6]

Monosodium glutamate (MSG) is another. Now sneaking into your food under its dozens of disguises (including monohydrate, L-glutamic acid, UNII-W81N5U6R6U, and monopotassium glutamate), it has been shown to cause severe impacts in various areas of the brain, leading to almost instant fatigue.[7]

And then there are the artificial sweeteners, like aspartame—and oh boy, where do we start with these? Numerous studies have uncovered negative cognitive, mental health, and neurological consequences linked with aspartame intake. Consuming large amounts of this artificial sweetener has been revealed to cause or intensify headaches and can even be a factor in increasing the risks for dementia and seizures.[8, 9, 10]

We must be incredibly careful not to consume these foods that can directly impact the brain. Consuming a lot of gluten is another example, and yes, gluten comes up *again*.

When exposed in the stomach to pepsin (an enzyme) and hydrochloric acid, gluten is degraded to a mix of polypeptides. These can cross the blood-brain barrier that separates the bloodstream from the brain. This barrier is there for a reason. The brain is highly sensitive to the wide variety of substances that gain entry to the blood, some of which can provoke undesirable effects should they cross into your amygdala, hippocampus, cerebral cortex, or other brain structure.

These polypeptides have been labeled *exorphins*. Exorphins, found not only in gluten but also in the casein in dairy, have an opioid-like effect on the brain, triggering the release of dopamine. Repeated exposure to them can lead to serious imbalance in the brain and a higher likelihood of depression and schizophrenia.[11]

At the very minimum, they immediately create foggy thinking, daytime fatigue, and physical sluggishness and are responsible for most of the afternoon energy slump so many people experience.

To support our mental energy (and mental health), we need to avoid processed foods and the awful chemicals they contain while also fueling the body with the nutrients that we know it needs to support mitochondrial function and power the brain with the energy it needs.

Hormonal Fatigue

Closely related to mental fatigue is the kind caused directly by an overstressing of the adrenals; aka *hormonal fatigue*. These sensitive glands are two endocrine organs that sit atop the kidneys, and the hormones they secrete assist in regulating metabolism, blood pressure, stress response, and other body functions essential for survival.

As we discussed earlier, stress is more acid forming than any food, and it's true! We absolutely need to manage our stress response. Experiencing stress over and over and over severely impacts the adrenals, and when they're triggered to release cortisol over and over and over, our energy plummets.

We haven't evolved to produce cortisol chronically like we do today. Think about humans in hunter-gatherer times. We experienced a stress response only in extreme circumstances, such as when a saber-toothed tiger approached our village, there was a famine, or a rival village attacked us.

In these extreme circumstances, the stress response is triggered, and we experience four immediate physiological responses:

- Blood sugar rises to deliver more glucose to the brain
- Blood pressure goes up to deliver more oxygen to your brain
- Blood becomes more prone to clotting (so that if a tiger attacked you, you'd be less likely to bleed to death)
- The amygdala becomes hyperreactive, becoming vigilant of every threat around you

The problem is, we are not only getting stress responses to tigers attacking once every few months or so. *We are activating our stress response all day, every day.* We do this with our e-mail inbox, social-media doomscrolling, our kids fighting, perceived money stress, social anxiety, work deadlines, missing the bus, what someone said on Twitter, the person who cut in front of the line at the store, the news . . . you get the picture.

This stress response is helpful in the short term while a tiger is nearby, but it's devastating when it's chronic, all day and every day. When the amygdala is overstimulated, your blood sugar and blood pressure go up, and fatigue sets in almost instantly. And when we constantly put pressure on the adrenals to pump out more and more cortisol, 24/7, the constant fight-or-flight mode of cortisol swirling through our body is absolutely devastating to our energy.

So we have this emotional, stress-response impact on the adrenals. But there is a just-as-impactful dietary side too, and you won't be surprised to hear that DIA is the culprit.

Studies show that when we are in a state of DIA, it triggers the adrenals to overproduce even more cortisol.[12]

And the cruel twist of nature? Not only does DIA increase cortisol production, but overproduction of cortisol drives blood pH down to make you more acidic! It's another vicious cycle. And when fatigue and emotional stress often cause people to reach for sugar, caffeine, comfort (processed, packaged) food, breads, pastas, and treats, the vicious cycle gets even deeper and wider.

We need to break this cycle, and in the Alkaline Life Plan we most certainly do! You can do it easily and quickly from a dietary perspective; and from an emotional, stress-response perspective, we'll set some foundations for you that will make a huge impact quickly and give you tools to help support you with the ongoing stresses of life.

Inflammatory and Acidic Fatigue

Finally, we're at the fourth cause of fatigue. Based on everything we've covered so far, DIA causes fatigue-lowered functioning in every major system in the body. When the state of DIA causes lower liver function, lower kidney function, mitochondrial dysfunction, slower metabolism, stress to adrenals, gut imbalance, stress to the thyroid, and insulin resistance—along with the huge energy required to buffer acidity and raise blood pH from acidic back up to the safe zone—it's clear to see how DIA could be the root cause of fatigue.

When there's a consistent release of inflammatory cytokines (proteins) in the blood, the body undergoes a huge amount of stress as it tries to cope. This can cause chronic fatigue, especially when disease activity is high, or low-grade inflammation remains for a long time. Chronic inflammation leads to reduced cellular energy availability and encourages insulin resistance. It also causes sleep disturbances and a loss of restorative, deep sleep, which of course increases feelings of fatigue.[13]

To put it simply, if our diet induces acidosis and inflammation, we will experience fatigue. That is a guarantee. And once we remove the acidosis, fatigue is replaced with amazing, abundant, all-day energy.

ELIMINATING FATIGUE AND GETTING ENERGIZED CAN BE ONE OF THE EASIEST AND QUICKEST GOALS TO REACH

Malnourishment fatigue, mental fatigue, hormonal fatigue, and inflammatory fatigue are all interlinked, and the solution is simply to get your body out of the all-day, every-day acidic safe zone.

As you can imagine, the one system that is perhaps most important to all of this is your digestive system. So much of your energy production, or lack thereof, is rooted in the gut (your second brain).

To achieve wonderful, sustained energy, we need to have a balanced, thriving digestive system. So let's get into that next.

20/80 ACTIONS FOR FIGHTING FATIGUE

Action One: Get Rid of Candida

Excess candida in the digestive tract is a very, very common cause of fatigue. During your Alkaline Life Plan, you will, over time, naturally reduce the acidic foods that contribute to candida (such as gluten, yeast, and sugar), but a rapid way of killing candida is *coconut oil*. The caprylic acid in coconut oil is proven to kill many strains of candida, including *Candida albicans*.[14] An overgrowth of candida in the gut causes loss of nutrient absorption, inflammation, toxic overload, and immune system stress. All of these, individually and together, contribute to feelings of fatigue.

Candida overgrowth also leads to the production of the acidic toxin acetaldehyde in the digestive tract, which is known to cause fatigue, brain fog, and migraines.

Action Two: Fight Inflammation

The most powerful, yet simple way of fighting inflammation is to have a homemade turmeric-and-ginger tea or latte as part of your morning routine. These drinks (page 254) contain around a centimeter each of turmeric and ginger root, which have a rapid and potent impact on inflammation. You can double down on this with a curcumin supplement too.

Action Three: Encourage Proper Waking Cortisol Levels

The energy you feel throughout the day is largely dictated by your waking cortisol levels. If your waking cortisol is out of whack, it creates a cycle throughout the day where you never feel energized. The whole of the Alkaline Life Plan contributes to ensuring proper cortisol balance, but there are a few simple steps you can take to support this (which will also hugely help your sleep quality too).

First, upon waking, as quickly as reasonably possible, get outside and get sunlight. The natural light hitting your eyes triggers an essential release of cortisol.* Next, make sure you *never* look at a phone, tablet, or other electronic device the first thing in the morning. The dull light from the device is enough for your eyes to think that it's sunlight and start to produce the additional cortisol you need in the morning, but it's so dull, you'll produce nowhere near enough. And finally, no caffeine for the first 45 minutes of the day. Caffeine triggers the adrenals to produce a little cortisol, which then disrupts the proper balance of cortisol production from your circadian rhythm.

Action Four: Adequate Magnesium

Magnesium is not only essential in supporting the body's ATP production, but it also helps support sleep quality, so it's a double bonus. From a supplement perspective (page 87), magnesium glycinate will help your body with ATP, and magnesium threonate is especially well absorbed by the brain and supports mental energy. And, just as important, it is proven to improve sleep quality.

---

* It's important to note that I am not advocating that you stare directly at the sun! That is not a good idea. Instead, simply be outside in the morning sunlight, facing approximately toward the sun. Never look directly at the sun in a way that causes discomfort or pain. It's also important to note that you can't achieve this benefit by looking through a window, as the glass filters many of the important wavelengths.

· CHAPTER 12 ·

Digestive Healing

When we think of the digestive system, we think of acid. And yes, acid plays a big role, but this tells only a tiny part of the story. I know that a question on a lot of people's minds (and maybe yours) is:

"If the stomach is acidic, what's the point in eating alkaline?"

At first glance, this is a logical question to ask, because indeed, if everything is dropping into this big pool of acid and turning to sludge, then what difference does it make if a food is alkaline or acidic in the first place?

It turns out, the answer is: *a lot.*

All digestive imbalance and the resulting health challenges, including gut dysbiosis, gastroesophageal reflux disease (GERD), gastroenteritis, leaky gut, bloating, pain, and irritable bowel syndrome, almost exclusively result from the diet. And in most cases, these are due to the acidosis that the poor diet creates.

Maybe you don't associate your gut with your goals, like overcoming fatigue, skin conditions, allergies, low libido, or foggy thinking, but you absolutely should! Your digestive system overlaps with every single one of the other Five Master Systems—the immune, endocrine, detoxification, and pH balancing systems.

Your gut produces and manages dozens of your most important hormones, such as those weight-loss hormones leptin and ghrelin we discussed in Chapter 10, and 22 other hormones that aid digestion, proliferate cells, regulate proteins, stimulate and release energy, and control appetite.

When it comes to your cognitive health, your gut is home to the largest concentration of mood-altering neurotransmitters like serotonin. We tend to think that anything to do with mood is housed in the brain, but 90 percent of the body's serotonin is housed in the digestive tract. In fact, tons of studies have shown a strong link between gut health and mood disorders.[1, 2]

Even your immunity is mostly controlled by your gut—it's where 70 percent of the cells that make up your immune system live!

The bottom line is: if you want abundant health, you must balance your digestive system, and it all starts with that relationship between alkaline and acid.

THE ESSENTIAL ROLE OF ALKALINITY IN THE GUT

Your stomach is *not* a big pouch of acid waiting for food to drop in, fizzle away, and then you're done. It just doesn't work like that. Instead, *most of your digestive system is alkaline!*

It seems counterintuitive, but stick with me here. I promise I will keep this as quick and simple as possible as we dig into the science of the gut.

The Dance between Alkaline and Acid

Digestion doesn't actually start in your stomach. It begins as soon as food or drink enters your mouth. Immediately saliva and mucus and a handful of other enzymes in the mouth and throat start preparing the food and sending signals to the digestive system.

When the food hits the esophagus, the release of gastrin is triggered in the stomach, which triggers the release of hydrochloric acid (HCl).

The newly released HCl moves the pH of the stomach from its baseline level of pH 5 to 6 (only mildly acidic) down to a stronger acidity of around pH 4. At pH 4 the food can be easily broken down and any bacteria destroyed.

The stomach creates hydrochloric acid on demand to match the food or drink you've consumed and knows how much to create from the messages it has received from the mouth and esophagus.

Step One: The Stomach Produces Acid on Demand to Match the Food You Consume.

This is important: the more *alkaline forming* a food is, the more acid the stomach produces. Wait, what? Why? Remember, the stomach has to be at pH 4 to facilitate proper digestion. So when something alkaline forming comes along, it needs to produce *more* hydrochloric acid to bring the pH down. The stomach is very mildly acidic until we eat something, and then the volume of HCl it produces will vary depending on what we eat.

So if we eat lots of alkaline-forming foods, there will be more acid. But if we eat lots of strongly acidic foods, the stomach doesn't get the trigger to produce more acidity, because the pH is already low due to the acidity of the foods eaten.

Makes sense, right? The stomach needs to have the pH lowered, so if there's an alkaline substance coming in, it needs to trigger the release of *more* hydrochloric acid than if there's a pH 3 soda coming in—when it wouldn't need to release any more HCl at all.

More acid production is what we want! Even if you have GERD, this is what you want! Again, I know, it sounds counterintuitive, but stick with me. We *want* the stomach to produce hydrochloric acid. This acidity is a *good* thing! Because whenever the stomach produces the acid, it also produces a corresponding amount of highly alkaline sodium bicarbonate ($NaCOH_3$).

Step Two: The Stomach Produces Sodium Bicarbonate ($NaCOH_3$) in Response to the Hydrochloric Acid (HCl) It Has Produced.

The more acid your stomach produces, the more alkalinity it produces. Sodium bicarbonate production is *essential*. The sodium is passed into the bloodstream for a number of important functions and plays the crucial role of *raising* the pH of the semi-digested food back up to an alkaline pH so that it can be properly processed in the next phase of digestion, in the duodenum and small intestine.

This is critical for a healthy gut. You absolutely *need* this NaCOH$_3$ production, and the only way it happens is when HCl is produced.

In other words, eat alkaline to make the acid, which makes the alkaline!

The pH Levels of Each Stage of Digestion

Eating alkaline isn't about making your whole body more alkaline! It's about providing your body with the tools it needs to effortlessly *maintain* delicate pH balances. These are the ideal pH levels at each stage of the digestive process:

Throat/Esophagus: 6.8
Stomach: outside of digestion, pH 5 to 6; upon digestion, 3 to 4
Duodenum (small intestine phase I): 7 to 8
Jejunum/Ileum (small intestine phases II and III): 8
Large intestine (colon): 5.5 to 7—and the semi-digested mixture of food and digestive enzymes, known as *chyme*, which remains here during excretion, has a pH of 7 to 7.5.

An overly acidic diet causes the wrong parts of the digestive system to get too alkaline and out of balance. The Alkaline Life creates the homeostasis and balance your body needs everywhere—from the acidic stomach to the neutral esophagus, the alkaline small intestine, and the acidic large intestine.

Without the Acid, We Don't Get the Alkaline

Having an acidic stomach is critical for health, critical for alkaline balance, and critical for digestion—but it must be delicately balanced. And we can guarantee a balance by eating alkaline-forming foods.

NO MATTER YOUR GOAL, YOUR GUT PLAYS A ROLE

Having too much or too little HCl produced by the stomach contributes to the following symptoms, plus so many more: candida of the esophagus, diverticulosis, GERD, acid reflux, gastritis, peptic ulcers, dyspepsia, enteritis, colitis, short bowel syndrome, malabsorption, celiac, appendicitis, functional colonic disease (IBS, Ogilvie syndrome), Crohn's disease, abdominal angina, infectious diarrhea, rectal prolapse, anal fissures and abscess, hepatitis, cirrhosis, fatty liver, liver failure, liver abscess, gallstones, pancreatitis, and autoimmune conditions (such as Hashimoto's thyroiditis, rheumatoid arthritis, Graves' disease).

It completely messes with your body's immune system (hence the autoimmune conditions) and disrupts your hormones, leading to stress and imbalance in the thyroid, adrenals, parathyroid, hypothalamus, pituitary, pancreas, ovaries, and testes. The endocrine system manages hormones that regulate metabolism, growth and development, tissue function, sexual function, reproduction, sleep, and mood—and a compromised digestive system directly imbalances this.[3]

I can't emphasize this enough: you must have good, well-balanced digestion to have abundant health, and an acidic diet is the single most damaging thing you can do to this entire process.

Angela's Story

When I was 59 years old, I had absolutely terrible heartburn and digestive pain and had been on daily Nexium for 4 years. I had become reliant on it and would always keep some on me in case the acid reflux got really unbearable. At one time the pain was so intense that I fainted! I wasn't happy about taking any medicine that my body was reliant on, and when I asked my health professional what I could do to come off the tablets, she flippantly replied, "Just lose some weight." As if I hadn't been trying for several years!

I also had adrenal fatigue and was concerned that having an unhealthy body could lead to many ailments, including cancer. Being determined to turn my life around, I looked online for sound advice for weight loss in postmenopausal women, but there didn't seem to be any. And then I found the Alkaline Life Plan!

After following the Alkaline Life Plan for only a month or so, I was able to completely give up all tablets. I am now 35 kilograms [77 pounds] lighter, and at the age of 65, I am healthier than I've been in decades. I have taken up yoga, which I *love*, and I walk 35 to 40 kilometers per week, as I'm in training to walk 300 kilometers [186 miles] of the Camino Frances. It is such a dream to be able to do this, and I am now entirely self-motivated.

20/80 ACTIONS FOR DIGESTIVE HEALING

Action One: Weed, Seed, Feed

To replenish and rebalance your gut bacteria, you need to take it step-by-step. What you do *not* want to do is simply take a whole load of probiotic supplements and hope for the best. At best, this will be a waste of money. At worst, it will actually further unbalance your gut.

Step one is Weed. This is where you eliminate the causes of the gut imbalance and the foods that fuel the bad bacteria, namely, sugar, gluten, and processed foods. You should reduce and restrict them for at least two weeks.

Step two is Seed. This is where you consume naturally occurring probiotic-rich foods such as kimchi, sauerkraut, miso, and kombucha. These foods are slightly acid forming by nature, so we consume them consistently only for the two weeks that make up the *Seed* part of the plan. A supplement can also be used here, but it's only to supplement, not as the main source of the good bacteria.

Step three is Feed. This is where we taper back down on the fermented foods and add in lots more fresh vegetables that will help the body to naturally maintain its beautiful gut balance. We can still use fermented foods here and there, but it's for enjoyment now, rather than therapeutic.

Action Two: Hydrate Properly Every Day

We need to support the digestive system to help clear out all of that clogged-up, undigested matter in the small intestine. Dehydration contributes to this, and hydration clears it out. So many of us are walking around in digestive imbalance and are dehydrated. You cannot be healthy and dehydrated. Aim to consume at least 80 to 100 ounces of filtered water daily.

Action Three: Take Coconut Oil to Kill Candida

Candida overgrowth is one of the main causes of an unbalanced microbiome, causing inflammation to the gut lining; exacerbating bloating, gas, and discomfort; and impairing nutrient absorption—which leads to the production of acid wastes in the gastrointestinal tract, including acetaldehyde. Aim to consume approximately 1 tablespoon of coconut oil daily (more on *how* to do this in Part III).

Action Four: Take Psyllium Husks

A quick and easy win, psyllium husks give us both soluble and insoluble fiber, making them a fantastic fix for the digestive system. Simply mix a teaspoon of them per day of into water, give it a stir, and drink it.

The soluble fiber helps to lower LDL cholesterol, regulate blood sugar, and support healthy gut bacteria balance. The insoluble fiber doesn't dissolve in the water and passes through the digestive system intact, and so it aids in cleaning and helping remove the clogged-up waste in the small intestine. It also helps ease bloating, gas, and constipation, and it promotes proper, regular bowel movement.

The only little thing to remember is to drink an additional glass of water straight after, as the husks can also absorb a lot of moisture in the digestive system, leaving you a little dehydrated.

· CHAPTER 13 ·

Stronger Bones

We often think of our skeleton as the collection of bones that keep us upright. But we need the bones in our body for so many other functions than just the ability to stand.

Bones are made of two major components: a hard outer layer (called the *cortical bone*) and a spongy inner "matrix" composed of the bone cells *osteoblasts* and *osteocytes*, bone-resorbing cells called *osteoclasts*, and a mix of collagen, proteins, and minerals.

Because of the complex role and ingredients that make up the bone—*and* the unfortunate fact that as we age, we slowly lose the ability to rebuild and repair the bones—strengthening them is essential. And our diet is the primary way we can do this.

WHAT ELSE DO YOUR BONES DO?

Aside from simply keeping you upright and able to move and physically function (which is a big job in itself), your bones are also responsible for a host of other key functions in the body, including the following:

1. **Blood cell production.** Your bones are responsible for a process known as *hematopoiesis*. This is the creation of blood cells that takes place in the bone marrow. The production of new blood cells is critical to practically every function in the body either directly or indirectly, which is why we need to eat lots of lovely greens.

2. **Mineral storage.** The bones and teeth store up to 99 percent of all your body's calcium and are largely responsible for calcium metabolism too, ensuring that your calcium can be used and transported. We tend to think of calcium as important only for building bone strength, but it's also essential for ensuring muscles, nerves, and cells can work optimally.

   Phosphorus is also found in your bones and is needed for the growth, maintenance, and repair of all tissues and cells and to produce the genetic building blocks of DNA and RNA, as well as to help balance vitamin D levels, which is essential for strong bones.

   Feeling tired? I bet you never considered your bone marrow in the equation! Bone marrow supports the storage of iron in ferritin and is involved in iron metabolism, a deficiency of which is strongly correlated with chronic fatigue.

3. **Hormone regulation.** Your bones are responsible for assisting in the regulation of several important hormones. Bone cells release a hormone called *osteocalcin*, which assists in all manner of balances in the body, including blood sugar regulation, fat storage, and surprisingly, your fight-or-flight response.

   In 2020, researchers from Columbia University discovered that osteocalcin is even *more* responsible for regulating the fight-or-flight response than adrenaline release.[1] They quite cruelly measured this by tricking people into thinking they had to deliver a speech in front of an audience! They found that all of the measures of the fight-or-flight response, such as heavy breathing, quickening of pulse, and a spike in blood sugar, were caused by a rapid increase in osteocalcin.

BONE DENSITY AND DIET-INDUCED ACIDOSIS

There are perhaps more published studies to show the impact of DIA on bone density than almost any other health challenge. This was arguably the first area of study that really attracted a lot of attention and funding with regard to the alkaline diet and health. A PubMed search for "alkaline diet bone" gives over 1,400 studies. The data is clear: an acid-forming diet causes net bone loss, and an alkaline-forming diet supports bone strength.

The Amazing Dr. Frassetto

Dr. Lynda Frassetto of the University of California, San Francisco (USCF), was one of the pioneers of research into the connection between an alkaline diet and bone health. I owe her a great deal for bringing solid data around the regulation of acid-base balance and the dietary influences on it into the forefront. Her 2001 paper "Diet, Evolution and Aging"[2] was the first I read that made the connection of "humans suffering from the consequences of chronic, diet-induced low-grade systemic metabolic acidosis."

The randomized, controlled trials looking into diet-dependent acid load and the renal function that she published in May 2023 shows that she's still working hard to discover more about the importance of acid-base balance.[3]

To maximize our bone mineral density (BMD) to its fullest potential, we need to avoid acid-forming foods and consume lots of alkaline-forming foods. This instantly raises a question I get asked a lot: "Isn't dairy good for your bones?"

Erm. I hate to break it to you, but . . .

THE GREAT DAIRY DECEPTION

Almost every single one of my students in the Alkaline Life Club who has the goal of stronger bones or reversing osteoporosis comes into my world a little nervous. They know I'm going to say that dairy is acid forming, but they have also been told they need to eat and drink lots of it. We need the calcium for strong bones, right?

Correct. We do.

We need calcium, along with protein and collagen, magnesium, phosphorus, vitamin D, and potassium[4] for strong bones. These are all alkaline-forming nutrients that thankfully come wrapped in delicious ingredients.

But there are two important things to note here:

1. We've been led to believe that calcium is the only thing we need for strong bones.

2. We've been led to believe that dairy is the *only* source of calcium.

Neither of these myths are true. And what makes things worse is, dairy leads to *weaker* bones!

I know!

There have been dozens and dozens of studies that demonstrate this, including this one published in the *American Journal of Public Health*. The study was conducted over 12 years with almost 78,000 women and showed those who drank more milk (more than three glasses per day) had more bone breaks than those who rarely drank milk.[5]

Another cohort study of 96,000 men who were over 22 years old showed that the more dairy they consumed as teenagers, the greater risk they had for fractures as adults.[6]

How Many Vegans Do You Know?

Have you ever wondered why there are such high osteoporosis rates in the U.S. when according to the data, less than 6 percent of its population is vegan?[7]

If 94 percent of the population is consuming milk, cheese, and so on, how are there over 55 million U.S. citizens aged over 50 with osteoporosis and osteopenia?[8]

Most people are consuming more than enough dairy to get the RDI of calcium, but osteoporosis or low bone mass is still affecting a huge percentage of the population.

It's Not Just about Calcium In

Consuming calcium is only about 10 percent of the equation. The other 90 percent is ensuring we don't *lose* the calcium that's already in our body.

Our body is constantly shedding bone material (its fancy name: *bone resorption*) and building new bone from the building blocks we provide through our diet. This process is easily knocked off balance in an acidic diet.

If we eat an acid-forming diet, not only are we consuming very few of the building blocks of bones (alkaline minerals) to replace the bone resorption, but our body is also *removing* calcium from our bones to buffer the acidity. Double whammy.

Dairy is *not* the answer. Not only is the calcium from dairy poorly absorbed, but it severely stresses our body's pH buffering system to deal with the acidity caused by the dairy.

Dairy is a highly acid-forming food, largely due to lactose and D-galactose, and we lose more calcium (and other bone-essential alkaline minerals) than we gain.

And guess what happens if you keep on drawing calcium from the bones? They get much weaker.

THE BONES' WORST NIGHTMARE

Think about the standard modern diet: sugar, soda, gluten, cheese, milk, ice cream, alcohol, margarine, jams, pastries, donuts, coffee, pizza, chips, ready-to-eat meals, oven meals, microwave meals, takeout food, sweets.

It's no wonder that 55 million U.S. citizens have low bone density or osteoporosis.

We cannot consume a highly acid-forming diet and expect to have strong bone density. To repeat, the equation for stronger bones consists of more than just calcium *in*. You must focus even more on preventing the calcium *out*, including the net calcium loss from consuming dairy and other acid-forming foods.

We have to focus our diet on the alkaline-forming foods that are rich in the nutrients to support your bones and then reduce the acid-forming foods to prevent the body robbing those bone-essential alkaline minerals to buffer the acidity from the diet.

Helen's Story

My story starts well over 20 years ago, when I was diagnosed with having osteoarthritis in my left hip. I was in a very stressful job, working long hours. With my practice, my job, and a house to run with two children at home, I was running on empty and felt like I had no time for anything.

The final straw came when I started to get the shakes from coffee. I couldn't control my hands shaking, and this frightened me. I did lots of research on osteoporosis and wanted to better my life, and I knew it started with my body and mind.

Within several days of living the Alkaline Life, I felt so much better and my energy had returned. I was sleeping so well and waking up feeling refreshed. My mind was clear, and I felt focused.

The results kept on growing. I feel nourished, my skin is clear, my hair is shiny, my teeth are so white, and any aches I had, especially in my hands, are now completely gone. Even the brown spots on my hands have vanished.

And the osteoporosis? When my doctor ordered my bone and blood tests, he told me he had to check the results twice! My bone density had normalized, and my blood tests were perfect. I left his office feeling like I was on cloud nine, and still am. I am now 70 years, and everyone says I look 55.

20/80 ACTIONS FOR STRONGER BONES

Action One: Supplement Smart

There's a small, specific number of key supplements that can be a huge support for your bones. As I always say, supplements are there to supplement, and you *will* get all of these nutrients through your diet, but this little collective of extra boosters is a big help for your bones.

The goal is to get these nutrients daily:

—Collagen
—Vitamin D
—Magnesium
—Sodium

There are plenty of fantastic, hydrolyzed collagen supplements available now, and these also add around 10 to 11 grams of protein to your diet too. For vitamin D, I recommend a daily intake of between 3000 to 5000 iu if you're actively looking to increase bone density. For magnesium, again I recommend the glycinate.

Note: if you're having even only a single serving of leafy greens per day, you don't need to worry about vitamin K. Just half a cup of kale will give you 443 percent of your daily needs. And don't stress about overconsumption. Naturally occurring vitamin K is easily used by the body, and anything that isn't used is simply removed. It's synthetic vitamin K from supplements that has the stricter upper limit.

Sodium is an easy one. If you are not already using an alkaline mineral supplement that contains sodium, calcium, magnesium, and potassium, you can simply add ⅔ of a teaspoon of sodium bicarbonate to a glass of water. While sodium is not directly utilized in the production of bone, it is a very effective alkaline buffer that the body prioritizes for buffering dietary acids. It basically tops off your natural pH buffers and therefore prevents the body from drawing calcium from the bone to do this job.

Action Two: Have My Bone-Building Smoothie

This delicious smoothie contains the perfect ingredients for building bone strength; avocado for the healthy fats and antioxidants; kale for the vitamin K, magnesium, and calcium; pumpkin seeds for the phosphorus, magnesium, and protein; sesame seeds for the calcium; spinach for the vitamin C, K, and manganese; and coconut milk for more healthy fats.

You can find the recipe, alongside more bone-building breakfasts, lunches, and dinners at www.thealkalinelifebook.com/recipes.

Action Three: Move

Movement has a huge impact on your bone strength. It doesn't have to be overly intense exercise if you're just starting out. Even walking has a big impact.[9]

Walking isn't going to be the total solution forever, but it is a fantastic start. Another option if you're concerned about impact and stress is using a mini trampoline, or "rebounder."[10]

CHAPTER 14

Thyroid Healing

There are two major disorders of the thyroid: hyperthyroidism, where the thyroid is overactive, and hypothyroidism, where it is underactive. Both are symptoms of diet-induced acidosis. Up to 60 percent of those with thyroid issues are unaware,[1] and thyroid conditions will affect up to 20 percent of us during our lifetime.[2, 3]

Your thyroid is a butterfly-shaped gland that forms an important part of your endocrine system (the system of organs and glands that regulates hormone production). It's especially important in that it produces the master metabolism hormones that play a part in controlling practically every other hormone in your body.

In other words, an imbalance here can have far-reaching consequences.

The most important hormones regulated by the thyroid are:

- T3: Triiodothyronine (controls energy levels, temperature, metabolism, heart rate, and blood pressure)
- T4: Thyroxine (controls how the heart works, metabolism, health of the muscles and bones, and brain development)

These "master" hormones help control and regulate the glands and organs elsewhere in your endocrine system and the other hormones they produce, including insulin, estrogen, cortisol, and testosterone.

HYPOTHYROIDISM VS. *HYPERTHYROIDISM*

The simple way to remember the difference between hypothyroidism and hyperthyroidism is that *hypo-* means "underactive" (leading to slow, sluggish metabolism; weight gain; fatigue; depression), and *hyper-* means "overactive" (fast metabolism, excessive weight loss). There can be several reasons for either condition, but they all come back to DIA and chronic inflammation.

What Is Hyperthyroidism?

Let's start with hyperthyroidism. This is when the thyroid gland is overactive, producing too much thyroid hormone thyroxine (T4). Typically, you may have heard of this as Graves' disease, or having thyroid nodules or an inflamed thyroid gland (often called *thyroiditis*).

Symptoms include:

- A superfast metabolism and an inability to gain weight
- Sudden, unexplained weight loss
- Brittle bones
- Eye problems
- Atrial fibrillation
- Thin, brittle hair
- Excessive anxiety
- Red, itchy skin
- Excessive, unexplained bowel movements

Hyperthyroidism is far less common than hypothyroidism, but the symptoms can overlap. It is almost entirely a symptom of chronic inflammation, and making dietary shifts toward alkaline-forming and anti-inflammatory foods can bring fast and lasting results.

What Is Hypothyroidism?

Hypothyroidism is characterized most by sluggishness. It occurs when your thyroid produces too little thyroid hormone.

Recognizing that you have hypothyroidism can be difficult, because the symptoms are so often seen as a "thing" in and of themselves. For example, people see weight gain or lethargy as the problem in isolation; they don't think about what could be causing it. They may start consuming fewer calories, thinking this will help them lose weight, when really, it will do absolutely nothing except perhaps make their thyroid imbalance worse.

Symptoms of hypothyroidism include:

- Weight gain (and difficulty losing weight)
- Fatigue (physical and mental)
- Lethargy and depression
- Rough and cracked skin
- Hair loss
- Infertility
- Digestive issues, especially constipation
- Frequent colds and flu and generally lowered immunity
- Sudden, unexplained menstrual cycle changes

THE TIP OF THE ICEBERG

When our body has an acidic imbalance in one area, it's almost certain to have caused an imbalance elsewhere, with its own set of symptoms and challenges.

As we've discussed, if your thyroid is not producing enough T4, your body will create visceral fat cells, slow your metabolism right down, and then hang on to the fat cells for dear life. But the weight gain is just the start. The first outcome is that the excess visceral fat inhibits the body's ability to regulate blood sugar, and the body then must produce more and more insulin to keep the blood sugar in check. This leads to insulin resistance and stress on the pancreas, which now begins to lose its ability to utilize fat as fuel, meaning more weight gain.

As the ongoing up and down of insulin and blood sugar gets bigger and bigger, the more it happens—with bigger highs and bigger lows. And when blood sugar gets too low, the adrenals produce cortisol to help bring blood sugar back up.

This is a big problem. Chronically elevated cortisol now has its own impact. As we discussed in Chapter 3, this stresses your adrenals, leading to adrenal fatigue, and when the adrenals are impaired, they do not produce the correct volume of thyroid-stimulating hormones, leading to deeper hypothyroidism. A vicious cycle has started.

Furthermore, when our cortisol is elevated, the body goes into a state of low-grade acidosis,[4] leading to inflammation that immediately impairs thyroid function. Another vicious cycle.

We could go on and on here. The point is that one imbalance can easily cause another and create feedback loops that cause the vicious-cycle effect, where things really can spiral out of control.

But thankfully we can put a stop to it!

It's Just More Iodine, Right?

There's an obsession with iodine in the "thyroid circles." If you do a Google search for hypothyroidism now, I would bet that *iodine* is the most frequently appearing word. But iodine's effect is being massively overstated.

While it can be an *influence*, the overexaggeration of the impact of so-called high-goitrogenic foods causes most people to miss the big picture.

Isn't Kale Bad for the Thyroid?

It's frustrating to see the recent articles claiming that suddenly, anyone and everyone should now avoid cruciferous vegetables like kale and broccoli. I want to make this clear: cruciferous vegetables are ridiculously good for you—they are alkaline, antioxidant-rich, proven cancer fighters that contain an abundance of nutrients that are so important for your thyroid health, as well as the rest of your endocrine system.

So why, then, are some people saying to avoid them?

The fuzzy logic is because cruciferous vegetables such as kale, bok choy, broccoli, brussels sprouts, cabbage, watercress, and arugula contain substances that are goitrogenic (meaning they can lead to the formation of a goiter).

And substances that cause a goitrogenic reaction can inhibit iodine from reaching your thyroid—and the thyroid needs iodine for proper functioning. However, this risk is being hugely overblown.

You would have to eat a massive, dangerous amount of these foods all day, every day, and *also* have severe chronic iodine deficiency for this level of goitrogenic activity to even register with your body. The body *easily* copes with the goitrogenic foods we eat.

Research has not shown any link between these deliciously healthy vegetables and a detriment to thyroid health. The study most naysayers cite is actually a single-case study (one person) of an 88-year-old woman who had been eating 2 to 3 pounds (1.0 to 1.5 kg) of raw bok choy daily for several months.[5] Which is not a normal, healthy amount.

No other studies conducted have shown any link between cruciferous consumption and thyroiditis. In fact, deep-dive narrative reviews of the literature such as this study,[6] published in the journal *Nutrients*, found no risk posed by cruciferous foods, and could only conclude "consuming these foods as part of a varied, colorful, plant-based diet should not pose significant risks in healthy individuals, and, conversely, may be of great benefit."

In short, just ignore the hype. Cruciferous foods contain nutrients that are so important for thyroid health. They are alkaline, anti-inflammatory, antioxidant rich, cancer protective, heart protective, and essential for the heart, lungs, liver, kidney, and brain too.

THE ACTUAL CAUSE OF HYPOTHYROIDISM

Easily the most frequent cause of hypothyroidism is inflammation, which results in a condition known as Hashimoto's thyroiditis. Also known as chronic lymphocytic thyroiditis or autoimmune thyroiditis, it's where the immune system mistakenly attacks the thyroid gland, impairing its ability to produce hormones.

Inflammation is also a far more potent cause of iodine deficiency, as inflammation interferes with iodine absorption in the gut. Ironically, of course, cruciferous vegetables are very potent tamers of inflammation.

Acidity

A diet high in acid-forming foods creates the perfect environment for thyroid imbalance, both with hypo- and hyperthyroidism.

In a study published in the *American Journal of Physiology*, researchers demonstrated that when the body is in a state of chronic acidosis, thyroid function drops significantly. T3 and T4 production go down, and TSH (a biomarker of hypothyroidism) goes up significantly.[7] Elevated TSH is a problem in its own right, stressing the pituitary gland that produces it.

Oxidative Stress

When our antioxidant defenses are overwhelmed, the excess free radicals (reactive oxygen species, or ROS) directly impact our thyroid health. Remember, oxidative stress comes from too many acid-forming foods and too few alkaline-forming foods.

High levels of oxidative stress cause direct damage to the thyroid gland. The process of thyroid hormone production involves the body creating hydrogen peroxide, itself a ROS. Normally the thyroid then has the mechanisms to neutralize this, but when there is already an overwhelming amount of ROS from the diet, this process cannot happen properly and it causes damage to the thyroid.

Oxidative stress also affects the transport of thyroid hormones into cells and the receptors within them that the thyroid hormones bind to.

Poor Sleep

I could mention sleep in every chapter. It is so important. Much like hydration, sleep is one of those things we often just leave to chance. But you must make adequate, good rest a priority. It's an absolute necessity for your thyroid health.

Circadian rhythms and sleep quality influence the pituitary gland to release TSH, the hormone that regulates the release and volume of your thyroid hormones, thyroxine, and triiodothyronine.

In a study of over 140,000 postmenopausal women on poor sleep quality and sleep disturbance, an 11-year follow-up showed a significant link between poor sleep and increased risk of thyroid cancer.[8]

And men aren't off the hook! A 2021 study of 198,574 subjects showed that middle-aged men with obstructive sleep apnea had an increased risk of thyroid cancer.[9]

Poor sleep can also lead to poor immune response and poor digestion. Sleep is imperative in clearing out brain-degenerating toxins too. But again, we can apply those 20/80 principles to sleep, even if, like me, you have kids and pets and all sorts of other things going on that are swinging around like wrecking balls at a good night's sleep. You can still maximize the *quality* of your sleep to support you even when the quantity might be a little disrupted.

THYROID HEALTH IS ESSENTIAL

Thyroid health is not just about the thyroid. It is essential in the function of so many other organs and processes in the body. From our digestive system to our cognitive health and from our weight to our energy, we need a healthy, fully functioning thyroid for all of it.

While you may not have thought about your thyroid when considering your personal health goals, when you look at what we have touched on in this chapter with regard to weight, digestion, cancer, fatigue, and type 2 diabetes, you can see that practically no matter your goal, you need to support your thyroid function. And this is especially true if you have an inflammatory condition, such as autoimmune.

And because thyroid health plays a huge role in our immune function, this is where we're heading next.

Denise's Story

In 2009, I was suffering with thyroid disease, osteoarthritis, depression, unrelenting fatigue, and a 40-pound weight gain. I was literally hungry (pun intended) for information that would support my belief in the detrimental effects of sugar and the medicinal benefits of plant-based eating.

When I discovered the Alkaline Life, I never looked back. It completely changed my relationship with my body and with food. I was empowered to make mealtime the sacred ritual it remains today, where it nourishes me and supports my energy.

Now at 71 years old, my life is one of joy, vigor, and immense gratitude. The weight has gone, my energy is sky-high, my thyroid has normalized, and I am no longer depressed. My sleep is now wonderful and refreshing, which was previously such a problem for me. It has boosted my energy so much.

I have returned to my creative and physical passions and have been able to return to my job as a dance teacher, choreographer, and costumer. This is something I thought I had said good-bye to for good. I have also been able to return to yoga and hiking, and even skiing!

20/80 ACTIONS FOR THYROID HEALING

Action One: Drink a Turmeric-and-Ginger Latte in the Morning

This action is powerful for practically every health goal, but especially so for any thyroid, inflammatory, or autoimmune condition; a digestive imbalance; or just your liver, your kidneys . . . look, it's great for everything! This is something I recommend to everyone as part of their morning routine. I've included two recipes in this book (page 254), and I urge you to start making these drinks each day.

Action Two: Add Selenium

Selenium is an essential mineral that is *so* important for the thyroid and helps in the production of thyroid hormones. However, so many of us are deficient! Simply including 1 to 2 Brazil nuts per day will easily get you to your recommended daily levels of selenium.

Action Three: Snack on Nuts and Seeds

Healthy, quick, and easy alkaline snacks are a bonus no matter what, but if you want to support your thyroid, the zinc, iron, vitamin E, copper, and healthy fats that you find in nuts and seeds such as almonds, pumpkin seeds, sesame seeds, sunflower seeds, and Brazil nuts are incredible for the thyroid (and a great way to get that selenium too!).

Action Four: Get a Daily Dose of Vitamin D

Vitamin D is critical to thyroid health, so get yourself outside for a dose of sunlight every day *or* make sure you're supplementing with at least 2000 to 3000 iu of vitamin D daily.

· CHAPTER 15 ·

Boosting Your Immunity

If you frequently catch coughs, colds, flu, respiratory infections, and indeed, are concerned about any SARS virus, applying even the most basic principles of the Alkaline Life will help you to increase your immunity. Immunity is built in the gut, and it thrives with the nutrients that delicious alkaline foods provide—such as antioxidants, anti-inflammatories, vitamins, minerals, and compounds like sulforaphane and glutathione. Furthermore, the most acid-forming foods, like sugar,[1] gluten,[2] alcohol,[3] sweeteners,[4] and food chemicals[5] have been *proven* to suppress immune function.

Poor immunity is a direct result of DIA, and when immune function is low, we need to address this rapidly, as it's a precursor to so many other conditions. Not to mention that we don't want to catch every bug going around!

THE IMMUNE SYSTEM

Your immune system is an interactive network of organs, cells, and proteins that protect the body from viruses and bacteria or any foreign substances. It works to neutralize and remove these foreign invaders.

Of the Five Master Systems (immune, detoxification, endocrine, digestive, and pH balancing), the immune system is probably the most "behind the scenes." When it's working properly, you don't even know it's quietly protecting your body 24/7, going about its business and constantly asking everything that enters your body, "Hey! Are you supposed to be here?"

Whether or not the foreign organisms cause disease is decided by the integrity of your immune system. For example, if it's working well, germs come in and are recognized as intruders, and the body expels them. But when you have an under- or overactive immune system, things can go wrong, with a detrimental effect on the rest of the body.

If your immune system is underactive, you're more likely to suffer from colds and flu, of course. But more seriously, it can lead to severe infection, nervous system damage, and more. And of course, if your immune system is overactive, autoimmune diseases such as Hashimoto's, rheumatoid arthritis, and chronic fatigue are more likely to kick in.

If the other Master Systems—especially the endocrine, digestive, and pH-buffering systems—are out of balance, inflammation (the leading cause of an imbalanced immune system) increases.

It doesn't take a doctor, rocket scientist, or immunologist to tell you that eating badly, drinking excessively, not getting enough sleep or exercise, and living an unhealthy life will weaken your immunity. When you treat your body badly, you always catch more colds and flus, and feel run down. On the other hand, if you nourish and support your immune system, you stand a better chance of protecting yourself more effectively.

The Three Lines of Immune Defense

There are three lines of defense in your immune system:

1. *Physical and chemical barriers.* Physical barriers include your skin and mucous membranes, and chemical barriers include stomach acid and enzymes in your tears and saliva.

2. *Innate immune system.* Every cell in your body is primed to make interferons—antiviral molecules—when they detect an intruder. These immune cells start making their own antiviral molecules to stop the virus from replicating. The process produces cytokines (a type of protein), which cause fever and inflammation of the tissues. When these cells recognize they have been infected, they try to kill themselves off to protect you. White blood cells, also known as natural killer cells, are part of this first line of defense. They simply work to detect infected cells and kill them off.

3. *Adaptive immune system.* This takes a few days to ramp up. The adaptive system is made up of white blood cells such as T cells that try to kill infected cells, and B cells that produce antibodies that either neutralize the intruder or cover it with a substance so the T cells can recognize and kill it.

We need to support all three lines of defense through our diet and lifestyle choices.

HOW DIA IMPACTS THE IMMUNE SYSTEM

It should be no surprise, but eating an acidic, inflammatory diet is terrible for the immune system. The foods that cause chronic, diet-induced metabolic acidosis directly impact all three stages of the immune system.

Sugar

Sugar causes our blood glucose levels to rise and activate an enzyme known as *protein kinase C*. This has been linked to weakened immune response, particularly in white blood cells called *neutrophils*, whose job it is to travel, "eat," and subsequently destroy invading microorganisms. Sugar also affects cells called *phagocytes*, which are responsible for destroying bacteria and other foreign particles invading your body.

And artificial sweeteners are no better. Sucralose has been shown to affect the gut microbiome, which is where so much of the immune system is housed. A 2008 study showed a twofold decrease in the number of beneficial bacteria in the microbiome after consuming sucralose.[6]

High blood sugar is associated with the inability of immune cells to properly "tag" foreign pathogens so they can be destroyed and removed from the body.[7]

Gluten

We don't need to dive deep back into the effects of gluten again (see Chapter 5), but when we consider how pro-inflammatory it is, how it leads to leaky gut and bacterial imbalance, and how seriously acid forming it is, we can appreciate how awful it is for the immune system.

Food Additives

Additives such as artificial flavors, colors, preservatives, and stabilizers can be incredibly stressful to the liver, which is an important part of the immune system.

We've already touched on sucralose and artificial sweeteners, but artificial and natural colors and flavors, additives like MSG, and preservatives like phosphoric acid and PFAS can cause incredible stress to the liver and gut balance.[8]

Recent studies have demonstrated that the consumption of artificial sweeteners and dietary emulsifiers can alter the gut microbiome, resulting in intestinal disturbance and inflammation.[9] MSG can interfere with the normal functioning of your thymus and spleen, preventing them from producing enough lymphocytes to fight off infection.[10] Studies have also shown that intake of excessive phosphoric acid, an additive that until recently flew under the radar, can impact bone health and heart disease.[11]

What about "Natural" Flavors and Colors?

So, back in the day . . . in a past life . . . I used to work for a big beverage company. I was the innovation manager at the time, trying to bring some healthy beverages to their range (I worked on a never-to-be-launched breakfast smoothie for quite some time—it could have changed the world!). This meant I spent a *lot* of time working with the scientists and chemists to formulate new drinks and flavors, and I can tell you that "natural" colors and flavors are *not* natural. They are just as unnatural and unhealthy as your regular colors and flavors, and in many cases, they are actually worse.[12, 13]

Simple rule: do not believe the labels of any packaged foods!

HEALING THE IMMUNE SYSTEM WITH ALKALINE-FORMING FOODS

Supporting the immune system is not just about warding off coughs, colds, and viruses. A fully powered immune system is essential to all the other systems in the body. It needs to be in balance and thriving.

If you'd like to compile a list of the most *immune-healing foods*, refer to Chapter 2. These contain alkaline minerals such as zinc, magnesium, potassium, and antioxidants such as vitamins C, D, and E, the carotenoids and flavonoids, and those essential omega-3 fats.

To support the immune system, we have to get the gut flora back in balance, and we have to get the inflammation out. All of this is done with those Triple-A foods: alkaline forming, anti-inflammatory, and antioxidant rich.

Cali's Story

Having struggled for over a decade with my health, including multiple issues ranging from my weight to a struggling immune system, the alkaline lifestyle is the only thing that has managed to give me what I need. I feel fantastic!

I've lost 21.1 kilograms [46 pounds], I have gone down three dress sizes, and I've completely changed the way I eat. It's amazing how good I am feeling and how much healthier I am looking. There are so many benefits I feel now, like no bloating, improved skin and hair, improved energy levels, and improved focus—and I never get sick any more with coughs and colds!

But for me, perhaps the best part is that my husband is two weeks into doing the alkaline protocols too, and I have not seen him with this much energy and positivity since I first met him 13 years ago. He is buzzing, and it is so awesome for me to see him like this. A fabulous result of this way of eating for him is that he now has no heel pain at all! He has had major issues with his heels to the point that every doctor he had seen said he needed surgery. The anti-inflammatory nature of eating alkaline is clearly working.

20/80 ACTIONS FOR IMMUNE BOOSTING

Action One: Take the Immune-Boosting Super Shot

This healthy shot is simply juiced beet, ginger, and turmeric. It provides a huge hit of the most powerfully anti-inflammatory, immune-boosting, alkaline, antioxidant-rich ingredients in one fiery, delicious shot.

Action Two: Have Some Broccoli Sprouts

I know it sounds a bit odd, but if you can grow your own broccoli sprouts and include even just a handful each day, this will do more for your immune system than practically everything else combined. Broccoli sprouts contain the essential immune compound sulforaphane at huge levels (up to 100 times more than in the mature broccoli plant). The extra bonus here is that boosting sulforaphane levels in the body helps to boost its levels of glutathione too (your "master" antioxidant). I've created a guide to growing broccoli sprouts for you at www.thealkalinelifebook.com/sprouts.

Action Three: Have Some Raw Garlic

Garlic is great for the immune system, because it contains allicin, a proven antiviral, antimicrobial, and antifungal. However, much of the allicin is destroyed when garlic is heated. Getting your garlic raw, therefore, is a fantastic and potent immune booster. Consider adding raw garlic to your blended soups, dips, sauces, dressings, and even your alkaline smoothies.

· CHAPTER 16 ·

Tackling Type 2 Diabetes

Type 2 diabetes affects millions of people worldwide. In the U.S. alone, over 37 million people have a type 2 diabetes diagnosis, and it's estimated that a further 96 million people have prediabetes.[1]

Unmanaged type 2 diabetes (T2D) can have devastating consequences, including kidney failure, vision loss, amputations of the limbs and feet, nerve damage, and even ultimately death. It's one of the most common "foundational diseases" that dramatically increases the risk of a host of other serious conditions. Several studies have shown that following a T2D diagnosis, all-cause mortality risk increases by up to 3.4 times, and atherosclerosis and cancer are significantly far more likely with a T2D diagnosis.

In fact, Alzheimer's disease, kidney disease, nerve damage, eye damage, and mental health can all worsen with type 2 diabetes. It's not pretty. But it is completely avoidable.

Right now, I want you to know the good news: T2D is completely reversible through diet and lifestyle changes.

When you follow the Alkaline Life Plan, you can reverse T2D, get off insulin, and receive a whole host of other benefits along the way.

T2D AND DIA

Type 2 diabetes occurs when the body produces an insufficient amount of insulin or fails to effectively utilize it. As a result, glucose levels remain abnormally high in the bloodstream and can lead to serious damage to blood vessels, nerves, and immune system.

There's a *lot* of complexity behind the scenes, but it's simple to see how an acid-forming diet of processed foods, junk food, sweets, sugars, gluten, and additives could lead to the major issues behind T2D: too much glucose in the blood and insufficient capacity to produce the insulin to control and deal with it.

The Role of Diet-Induced Acidosis in T2D Risk

First, there are the three most obvious ways in which DIA contributes to increased T2D risk:

- **Direct impact on blood sugar and insulin.** We know that sugar and gluten are the most acid-forming foods in the SMD and that these both wreak havoc on our blood sugar, driving it higher and higher and causing the body to produce more and more insulin to try to manage it. As we discussed in Chapter 5, the amylopectin A in modern gluten-containing grains drives blood sugar up like nothing else. Which leads us to . . .

- **Inflammation impact.** Foods in the SMD are not only also terribly pro-inflammatory but also create an environment in the body where inflammation quickly gets out of control. Chronic inflammation is particularly troublesome to insulin regulation, as it damages the beta cells the pancreas makes that are responsible for producing insulin. Inflammation in fat cells also contributes to insulin resistance, since when the fat cells are inflamed, they are unable to respond to insulin and can't take up the glucose from the bloodstream as easily. Which leads us to . . .

- **Excess weight impact.** As we saw in Chapter 10, DIA
  causes weight gain in numerous ways, and this increases
  T2D risk substantially. Hundreds of studies have linked
  body mass index (BMI) to an increased risk, and it makes
  sense. With an increased BMI comes a greater risk of digestive imbalance, poorer liver and kidney function, increased inflammation, hormone disruption, and pancreatic stress. While having your BMI in the "healthy" range
  is not a guarantee you won't develop T2D, increased
  visceral fat is clearly a huge risk factor.

And Then There Are the Sneaky Ways . . .

You'll know from what we've discussed so far that an acid-forming
diet creates all of the conditions we've just mentioned, making it a
blueprint for insulin resistance and diabetes.

However, diet-induced acidosis can also increase diabetes risk
in several more insidious ways:

- Being in the safe zone of diet-induced acidosis has been
  shown to alter the capacity for insulin to bind to its receptors. Disrupting this first stage of the insulin-signaling
  pathway results in reduced glucose uptake by muscle
  tissues and exacerbates the beta-cell function mentioned earlier.[2]
- Next we're back to the cortisol. It may seem like I'm paint-
  ing the picture that cortisol is a bad thing, but it's really
  not. It's actually a fascinating and amazing hormone
  that's very important. However, *too much of a good thing*
  is never a good thing, especially when it comes to cortisol. Like so many things in our body, balance is needed.
  And DIA puts cortisol out of balance all day, every day.[3]
  And when this happens, we lose a lot of our capacity to
  counterregulate insulin. As we know, in the safe zone,
  the adrenal cortex is stimulated to secrete more cortisol,
  and chronically elevated cortisol dramatically reduces
  the capacity of the body to regulate insulin.[4]

- Finally, remember adiponectin from Chapter 12? We know that acidosis suppresses adiponectin. Adiponectin isn't responsible only for assisting the body to access fat for fuel; it also functions as an insulin sensitizer. Low adiponectin means disrupted insulin balance and increased insulin resistance risk. Circulating levels of adiponectin, which functions as an insulin sensitizer, and low adiponectin levels have been associated with increases in insulin resistance risk.[5]

We have to remove the acidity and replace it with nourishing alkalinity.

THE SAFE ZONE OF DIA FUELS T2D

Study after study is finding that being in chronic, low-grade metabolic acidosis (DIA) fuels and exacerbates insulin resistance and drives up the risk of T2D.

In a 2020 study in *Nutrition Journal*, researchers studied 5,406 subjects with no prior history of T2D, insulin resistance, cancer, or kidney disease. They followed up with the subjects for 7.4 years, analyzing their diet, and documented 3,449 insulin resistance cases. They found that those in the highest quartile of acid-forming diet eaters had a significantly increased risk of insulin resistance and concluded that "diet-induced metabolic acidosis is associated with an increased risk of insulin resistance."[6]

A 2014 study published in *Diabetologia*, looking at a cohort of 66,000 women, found similar results. Those who were in the highest 25 percent of acidic diet eaters were at a significantly increased risk of type 2 diabetes.[7]

In fact, research dating back as far as 1952 has highlighted this link between DIA and insulin resistance.[8]

The good news is that by decreasing dietary acid load, we're removing the foods most associated with blood sugar spikes, inflammation, visceral fat cell formation, raised cortisol, and insulin resistance. The simple solution is to follow the Alkaline Life Plan!

20/80 ACTIONS FOR TACKLING TYPE 2 DIABETES

Action One: Drink an A.M. Green Juice

The nutrients in a green juice including spinach, kale, broccoli, tomatoes, bell pepper, carrots, and beets are absolutely *perfect* for supporting blood sugar and insulin balance while also healing and soothing the pancreas. This is the perfect elixir for preventing type 2 diabetes.

Action Two: Add Cinnamon and Coconut Oil to Your Breakfast Oats

Having oats at breakfast is not only great for fiber and beta-glucans (a polysaccharide that can support cholesterol management, the immune system, and blood sugar regulation), but by adding coconut oil and cinnamon, you take it to another level. Cinnamon and the MCTs in coconut oils are known to lower fasting blood sugar levels and improve uptake of glucose into cells.

Action Three: Squat after Meals

This one is a little out of left field, but a short burst of exercise after meals helps the muscles take up glucose from the blood for energy, resulting in better post-meal blood sugar levels. Squats are great because they engage large muscle groups, but taking a brisk walk can be just as effective.

· CHAPTER 17 ·

Curbing Cardiovascular Disease

Cardiovascular disease, atherosclerosis, cerebrovascular disease, and other associated diseases are the biggest causes of death in the developed world. If we want to live longer and with a fantastic quality of life, it makes sense that we need to avoid the biggest causes of death!

I want to make the important point here that between 80 and 90 percent of atherosclerosis is preventable through diet and life-style changes,[1, 2] and I believe the biggest change you can make is getting out of DIA.

There have been dozens of conclusive studies on diet-induced acidosis and atherosclerosis risk, with all of them finding that when we're in a state of chronic DIA, the risks for heart disease, high blood pressure, atherosclerosis, and stroke all increase.

- A 2020 review study published in the journal *Nutrients* found that "high DAL (dietary acid load) negatively affects cardiometabolic risk factors. This has particularly been confirmed in case of blood pressure—elevated SBP and DBP—and the prevalence of hypertension . . ."[3]

- A 2015 study published in the journal *Nutrition* involving research on 2,028 people found that "dietary acid load was significantly and positively associated with hypertension."[4]
- A 2019 systemic review study including over 306,000 individuals, published in *Nutrition, Metabolism & Cardiovascular Diseases*, found that there was "a significant positive association between dietary acid load and hypertension."[5]
- A 2015 study in *Hypertension Research* involving 31,590 adults over a 10-year period concluded, "higher metabolic acid load was associated with an increased all-cause and cardiovascular mortality in a healthy population."[6]

It's quite clear: *remove the acidosis, and the risk of the biggest causes of death significantly decreases.*

CHOLESTEROL IS VITAL TO LIFE

Many of us immediately associate cholesterol with heart attacks, or at the very least with a decline in health. We've been told over and over that if cholesterol goes up, your risk of heart disease goes up. Simple and linear—more cholesterol, more clogged up arteries, right?

This is what we've been told for decades. But the reality is that it's just not true. And the data is conclusive on this.

So, I want you to suspend any preconceived ideas you have about cholesterol and fat and their possible impact on your health. Just clear your mind for a bit!

WHAT IS CHOLESTEROL?

Cholesterol is a fatlike, waxy substance in the bloodstream. It can be good or bad, but one thing is for certain: your body absolutely needs cholesterol to function properly. If your levels drop too low, you put yourself at risk for many, many serious issues.

A 2020 study showed that participants with the lowest total cholesterol had a threefold increased risk of all-cause mortality in comparison to those who had healthy levels of total cholesterol.[7] Another study published in the *Journal of Epidemiology*, examining 12,334 individuals in Japan, found that low cholesterol was associated with an increased risk of death from stroke, heart disease, and cancer, while *high* cholesterol did not increase risk at all.[8]

Let's Get Clear on Cholesterol

Cholesterol travels in the blood in the form of lipoproteins (fat wrapped in protein), and there are two major categories of cholesterol: low-density lipoprotein cholesterol (LDL-C) and high-density lipoprotein cholesterol (HDL-C). These can then be broken down further into different particle sizes.

LDL-C is sometimes referred to as "bad" cholesterol. This is because it's the kind of cholesterol that causes plaque to build up inside your arteries and can lead to heart disease.

HDL-C, or the "good" cholesterol, is critical to life. It's essential for so many functions, including bringing the bad LDL-C from the bloodstream to the liver, where it can be removed from the body.

If you have only ever thought of your liver as the detox organ, it's important to know it also plays an important role in cholesterol synthesis. Your liver also removes LDL-C and regulates how much HDL-C is produced and circulating in your body at any given time. If your liver is out of whack and exhausted by processing sugar, preservatives, and chemicals from processed foods, this function suffers.

Where Does Cholesterol Come From?

There are two ways cholesterol appears in the body:

1. Your liver produces it.
2. It comes in from the foods you eat.

For the cholesterol we get from food, just like we have *good* fats and *bad* fats, and *good* salts and *bad* salts, there are, of course, foods that raise *good* cholesterol (HDL-C) and those that raise *bad* cholesterol (LDL-C). We need to be mindful of this and make sure we maximize one while minimizing the other.

It's also very important to **forget the outdated notion that any food that contains cholesterol is bad for your heart**. It's *far* more nuanced than that, and we'll get into why in just a second.

What Does Cholesterol Do?

Cholesterol plays so many important roles in your health. For starters, your body needs cholesterol to make vitamin D. Without cholesterol, you become quickly deficient in it, and low vitamin D status is associated with an increased risk of cancer,[9] immune disorders and low immunity,[10] osteoporosis,[11] and chronic fatigue.[12]

Cholesterol is also essential in regulating hormones as well as building new cell membranes and brain cells. Low cholesterol is linked to cognitive decline,[13] increased dementia risk,[14] and mood disorders.[15]

Without enough cholesterol, your entire system gets disrupted—it literally impacts almost every process in your body. Your cell membranes, which are made of cholesterol, couldn't function properly. And your body would no longer be able to make CoQ10, which is one of the most important and powerful antioxidants that helps convert food to energy, preserves cell health, and prevents oxidative stress (aging).

Cholesterol is also a component of bile, which is a substance your body needs to digest foods properly, uses in membranes to build new cells, and uses to help regulate many hormones, including estrogen, progesterone, cortisol, aldosterone, and testosterone.

THE TWO FORMS OF CHOLESTEROL

It's incredibly important to note that cholesterol comes in two forms:

1. Unesterified or "free" (UC)
2. Esterified (CE)

Whether cholesterol is UC or CE determines whether we can absorb it or store it.

This is important to consider, because most dietary cholesterol (cholesterol we eat) is in the esterified form (CE) and therefore is not absorbed by the body and is almost entirely excreted. That's right—*the cholesterol we eat does not contribute to the cholesterol levels in your body or to the numbers in your blood tests.*

The cholesterol that is *made in the body* is by far the most dominant source of cholesterol that you have floating around in yours.[16, 17] It is synthesized largely in the liver and essential for so many functions. You do not need to worry about dietary cholesterol. Focus instead on supporting your body to optimize and balance it.

LOVING YOUR LIVER

Rather than being worried about eating less cholesterol, we need to change our focus to eating the nutrients known to support liver function. This is a *far* more effective way of optimizing your cholesterol levels. The liver is not only responsible for producing and regulating the levels of cholesterol in your body, but it also distributes cholesterol throughout the body and is responsible for *removing it!*

With an optimally functioning liver, you are *far* more likely to have healthy, well-balanced, and optimized HDL and LDL cholesterol levels.

SCRATCHING THE SURFACE

There's a lot of depth to get into here with cholesterol, including the different types, the different tests, and so much more. You can find a free, deeper guide to cholesterol, its important numbers, and the tests you need at www.thealkalinelifebook.com.

For now, I want the big takeaways to be:

1. Cholesterol is essential to your health.

2. Your cholesterol levels are almost entirely a result of the cholesterol your body produces, not the cholesterol you eat.

3. The liver is essential in maintaining your proper cholesterol levels.

And Triglycerides?

Triglycerides, like cholesterol, get a bad rep but are absolutely needed in the body. And also like cholesterol, I don't want you to fear them. They are the most common type of body fat and are also made in the liver, sourced from our diet. And like for cholesterol, we depend on our liver for proper functioning, regulation, and use of them.

There are two main types of triglycerides—medium-chain (MCT), and long-chain (LCT). Both have to be regulated primarily by the liver, and like cholesterol, need to be optimized. In the correct balance, MCTs have been shown to have numerous health benefits, such as supporting weight management,[18] healing digestion,[19] fighting fatigue,[20] helping prevent Alzheimer's disease,[21] reducing epilepsy risk,[22] and of course helping to reduce cardiovascular and metabolic disease risk.[23, 24] LCTs are a great source of stored energy, are essential in absorbing certain vitamins, and play a role in the production of several hormones.

The body needs triglycerides for energy production, and it's critical that we maintain healthy levels. Foods that provide a source of MCTs and LCTs assist with this.

FOCUSING ON THE WRONG THINGS

For the past 60 years or more, we have been told that if we want to lower our risk of atherosclerosis, we need to eat less fat and cut cholesterol out of our diet. But the studies tell us we've been focusing on the wrong things the whole time.

Fat is not the problem, and neither is dietary cholesterol. In fact, it's quite the opposite. Healthy fats and cholesterol are essential for health and *reduce* the risk of atherosclerosis.

To lower our risk of atherosclerosis, and therefore cardiovascular disease, heart disease, and everything in between, we need to focus on consuming those foods that contain lots of healthy fats, nourish the liver, and avoid the acid-forming foods that put the body into diet-induced acidosis.

20/80 ACTIONS FOR REDUCING ATHEROSCLEROSIS RISK

Action One: Drink Liver-Loving Teas

So many beneficial micronutrients that can support the liver are absolutely *delicious* as teas! At the risk of sounding British, I always knew tea would be the answer. In all seriousness, nutrients beneficial for the liver include milk thistle (*Silybum marianum*), dandelion root, turmeric, ginseng, licorice, and ginger. These are all fantastic herbal teas, and they also contribute to your hydration (which is also indirectly beneficial to supporting the cardiovascular system).

Action Two: Add MCTs

MCT oils are flavorless, so you can add them to any meal or have them straight from the spoon. They're also well tolerated by people who have sensitivities to coconut and cannot have coconut oil. And for those who have gastrointestinal sensitivity to fats, MCT oil *powder* allows you to still get this vital nutrient without the discomfort. Aim for 1 tablespoon per day.

Action Three: Make Chia Pots or Chia Water

Chia seeds are an incredible source of both fiber and healthy fats, two of the most essential nutrients for cardiovascular health and cholesterol regulation. Make chia pots by simply combining 4 tablespoons of chia seeds with 1 cup of coconut milk. Stir, and put them in the fridge until the seeds have swollen up, and then serve with some coconut cream or yogurt and some berries. That will serve 2. Chia *water* is even easier—just combine 1 tablespoon of chia seeds per person and 1 cup of coconut water per person (or even just plain water), stir, and wait for the seeds to swell up. Then drink it down.

CHAPTER 18

Addressing Cancer

This chapter is a little different from the others. I thought long and hard about including a chapter on cancer. On one hand, cancer is such an important topic to address. The role of acidity in cancer risk is significant, and addressing this can bring huge hope. On the other hand, cancer is a very complex topic that, in essence, requires a separate chapter for almost every different type (breast, colon, pancreatic, lymphatic, and so on).

What I want to do over the next few pages is give you the big-picture role of diet-induced acidosis in cancer risk and the confidence to know that by following the Alkaline Life Plan, you can greatly reduce it.

If you have a current cancer diagnosis, I want to be clear: there's nothing in this chapter, or the book, that is in any way a cure. The Alkaline Life Plan is designed to put your body in the best possible position it can be to heal itself, rebalance, rebuild, and function optimally; and within that environment, your body will stand the best chance possible.

So whether you want to prevent cancer, support your body through cancer, or support your body through a treatment plan, the steps that I'm about to share will give your body the best possible conditions.

Cancer is devastating, affecting practically every single one of us either directly or through a loved one. It's the second most common cause of death in the Western world.

But the good news is, at *least* half of cancers are preventable. The American Institute for Cancer Research,[1] Cancer Research UK,[2] and the World Health Organization[3] all estimate the number of preventable deaths from cancer to be at least 40 to 50 percent or more. Cancer Prevention Europe puts the figure at 75 percent,[4] and the journal *Pharmaceutical Research* estimates the number to be 95 percent rooted in diet and lifestyle factors.[5]

Cancer is the term used to group over a hundred different diseases that arise from the uncontrollable division of cells. You hear me talk about health at a cellular level all the time. This is one of the primary reasons why.

So, what makes cells divide and grow in this abnormal manner?

Cancer is caused by changes to genes that control the way our cells function, especially how they grow and divide. Genetic changes that cause cancer can be inherited from our parents and can also arise during a person's lifetime because of errors that occur as cells divide or because of damage to DNA caused by certain environmental exposures.

When I say "environmental exposures," this can, of course, mean exposure to toxins and carcinogens that are completely out of our control. But I'm also referring to the preventable things we're in control of—namely, diet and lifestyle.

We can absolutely play a huge role in preventing cancer and supporting our body to fight it too.

Again, this is in no way saying any food or drink can "cure" cancer. There are many significant factors involved, and things become infinitely more complex once there's a diagnosis. However, the data tells us that there's a lot we can do to support the body to *prevent* cancer.

THE EFFECT OF AN ALKALINE ENVIRONMENT

I want to make sure we are clear on this, as there are a few myths and some confusion surrounding how impactful living alkaline can be on cancer. The less honest folks out there have used a well-known study from Otto Warburg back in 1931 to sell their alkaline supplements on the basis of the claim that "cancer cannot survive in an alkaline environment" (in fact, that is a direct quote from his Nobel Prize–winning study).[6]

So what is the truth here? The reality is that Warburg's research was brilliant and groundbreaking, but some are misrepresenting it. He wasn't studying the link between acid, disease, and foods to show the benefits of the alkaline diet. He was researching it to expand our understanding of cancer. His research is right—cancer can't live in an alkaline environment—but this is only relevant in vitro (i.e., in a test tube or outside of the body).

But it isn't as simple as this.

We can't re-create, through diet, the same conditions in the body as Warburg tested in his study. As we've covered, the body regulates the cells and organs at the exact pH they need to be—the stomach, pH 2 to 4.5; the duodenum and pancreas, pH 7 to 7.5; the small intestine, 7.4; the large intestine, pH 5.5 to 7; lymphatic fluid, 7 to 7.5; the gallbladder, 6.8 to 7.5; and so on.

By eating alkaline, the body won't then suddenly *go alkaline* everywhere! If it did, you'd die with a condition called *metabolic alkalosis*, and you would be in a lot of trouble.

While it's true that an acidic environment increases the risk of cancer and that eating alkaline is designed to help reduce that risk, I want to set the record straight about these myths and how all this plays into the alkaline diet.

You are not trying to re-create Warburg's in vitro environment.

Eating alkaline won't make your whole body "turn alkaline" and kill the cancer cells. When you "eat alkaline," you are giving your body an abundance of nutrients to do the best it can to fight disease. An alkaline diet supports the body in maintaining homeostasis, and within that balance, it will increase its ability to prevent cancer.

STUDIES ON DIET-INDUCED ACIDOSIS AND CANCER RISK

There are dozens of important studies that have shown that living alkaline and preventing overacidity are powerful with regard to preventing cancer. Here's just a small selection of the many, but this tells us we're onto something here.

- *Breast cancer.* A 2018 study published in *The FASEB Journal*, with the analysis of 49,731 women and 2,155 breast cancer cases, showed diet-induced acidosis to be a significant risk factor for breast cancer, especially post-menopausal.[7]

- *Colon cancer.* A 2021 case-controlled study published by Cambridge University Press in the journal *Public Health Nutrition* with 499 participants found that a higher dietary acid load was correlated with increased risk of colorectal cancer and colorectal adenomas.[8]

- *Bladder cancer.* A 2022 case-controlled study of 765 patients published in the *Multidisciplinary Cancer Investigation* journal found direct associations between dietary acid load and bladder cancer.[9]

- *Pancreatic cancer.* A 2021 prospective cohort study involving 95,708 adults found that dietary acid load is associated with an increased risk of pancreatic cancer.[10]

WHY IS DIA SUCH A RISK FACTOR FOR CANCER?

If we look at each of the biggest risk factors for cancer, you can see from what we've covered already in this book that living alkaline would be a fantastic way to lower your risk.

Inflammation is perhaps the biggest variable, and we know that DIA creates a huge amount of inflammation in the body. All the most acid-forming foods are pro-inflammatory, and all of the most alkaline-forming foods fight inflammation.

Similarly, we know oxidative stress drastically increases cancer risk, and DIA is like an oxidative stress factory. Being in the safe zone creates oxidative stress in the body 24/7, regardless of the stress caused directly from the acidic foods.

And then the inflammation and oxidative stress together lead to DNA and cell damage through a cascade of biological processes. Looking at just oxidative stress, ROS interact with DNA and cause multiple types of damage. For example, they can cause single- and double-strand breaks in the DNA structure, delete or insert extra DNA bases, or cause base modifications.

DNA damage can also interfere with the process of replication and transcription, leading to mutations, and it's these mutations that can ultimately lead to the development of cancer.

Again, we're scratching only the surface here, but all of this is a result of DIA.

In his review study "Examining the relationship between diet-induced acidosis and cancer,"[11] Ian Forrest Robey identifies eight additional pathways in which diet-induced acidity increases the risk of developing cancer, as follows:

- Increased cortisol (see Chapter 2)
- Tryptophan metabolism
- Insulin resistance
- Disrupted leptin and adiponectin (see Chapter 9)
- Increased insulin growth factor (IGF-1)
- Osteoclast activation
- Increased lactic acid

Again, a theme we keep revisiting in this book is: complex problem, simple solution. If we address our diet and remove the environment of diet-induced acidosis, these risk factors can disappear.

CANCER-FIGHTING NUTRIENTS

If we want to help prevent cancer, we need to avoid diet-induced acidity and provide our body with the cancer-fighting nutrients it needs. The Alkaline Life does this in abundance. Alongside the nutrients you may already know as cancer protective, such as vitamin C, folate, vitamin D, and selenium, you'll find the Alkaline Life Plan is rich in a wonderfully diverse range of nutrients that can also help reduce cancer risk. These include antioxidants such as carotenoids (beta-carotene, alpha-carotene, lycopene, lutein, zeaxanthin, astaxanthin), flavonoids (quercetin, kaempferol, genistein, anthocyanins), and, of course, specific polyphenols we focus heavily on such as curcumin, isothiocyanates (sulforaphane), and the tripeptide glutathione.

I truly believe that if one were to devise the perfect diet to reduce cancer risk, it would be the Alkaline Life Plan. It removes diet-induced acidosis, inflammation, and oxidative stress while fueling the body with the exact nutrients that have been most proven to help fight cancer and balance pH.

Simply put, the Alkaline Life is an incredibly powerful preventive measure. And if you have cancer, it will give your body a strong, balanced, healthy environment to support healing. So no matter what therapeutic path you choose to take, your body will be supported and nourished.

Trish's Story

I started the alkaline journey a year and a half ago, when I was diagnosed with bladder cancer. I was determined that there was a link between cancer and diet and started searching for answers, which landed me on the living alkaline path. There has been no turning back for me. I have lost 40 pounds and now have a clean bill of health, approaching age 60. The cancer is gone.

I am "living energized" and recently hiked to the top of Table Rock, which is rated very strenuous. In the past I would have never tried anything like that. I will be forever grateful for the coaching.

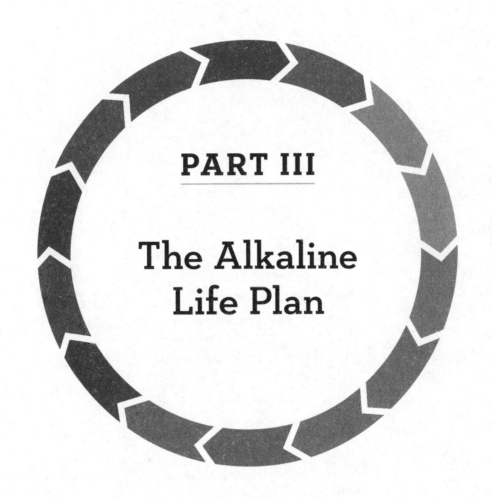

PART III

The Alkaline Life Plan

· CHAPTER 19 ·

A New Beginning

I'm so thrilled you're here. This is where things get exciting. You are now armed with all the knowledge to fully understand how to live alkaline and make it into a *lifestyle*. Because this is what we want, right? We don't want this to be temporary. We want lifelong, abundant health. We want to experience the joy that feeling our true health potential, all day, every day, brings. We want to wake up energized, feeling bright and focused and positive all day long—feeling strong and vital. This is what I want to bring to your life, and this next step is where I get really pumped up. This is where we get to work together.

This is my wheelhouse: *making it happen and making it stick.* And my superpower is making it easy, effortless, fun, achievable, realistic, and delicious.

I want you to see this as a new start. Remove any preconceptions you have. If you've tried to adopt a new, healthy diet in the past and failed, please forget that. Consign it to history, and know that any struggles you've had before *are not your fault.*

Remember, back on page 4, I said, "Results bring confidence. Confidence brings motivation. Motivation brings momentum. And momentum brings results."

This is what it's all about. And this is where we'll start.

WHEN DO WE START?

There really is no time like the present. But I understand that life can get in the way of this! Even so, I think it's important to realize that there is never the *perfect* time. There will always be a holiday, wedding, social event, birthday party, work function, weekend away, busy period, or *something* on the horizon.

My recommendation is that you start slow. Take it easy. Baby steps.

Here is how the Alkaline Life Plan works, and how I walk you through it in Part III:

- First, I walk you through the big-picture philosophy of the plan. I share with you my two cornerstone pillars that make up the foundation of the Alkaline Life Plan: Crowd Out the Bad and the Four Core Actions. If you ever get stuck, fall off track, or feel lost with your health, you simply come back to either of these foundational principles.

- Then we get into the 14-Day Plan with its daily actions; meal plans for breakfast, lunch, dinner, and snacks; and your hydration steps—plus your recipes, goals, and what you need to look out for.

- Finally, I get into the real-world questions that I know you might have about putting everything into practice and overcoming the hurdles that we all face when we start a new healthy-living plan. I know from experience that overwhelm is the biggest killer of motivation and action, so we keep this laser-focused on getting you the biggest results possible while setting you up for a lifetime of effortless health.

The Best Way to Start Is the Way That Works for *You*

You have two ways of approaching how you put this into practice.

You can start full throttle with the 14-Day Alkaline Life Plan, shopping for the ingredients the day before and jumping straight into Day One of the meal plan as soon as you wake up. This method will bring you the biggest results, fastest.

Alternatively, you can start even more gently and just apply the Crowd Out the Bad and Four Core Action fundamentals for a few weeks while you build your confidence and get up to speed, with a date firmly set in the diary for starting the more regimented 14-Day Meal Plan.

My recommendation is to do whichever you feel most comfortable with. It must feel right for you, and as I always say, *one size fits . . . ONE!*

As you read through Part III, you will intuitively know which way to go, and I encourage you to always trust your intuition.

Let's get into it!

At www.thealkalinelifebook.com, I've created an Alkaline Life pack for you to make this as implementable as possible. It contains a summary of everything we're about to cover, plus the Meal Plan, recipes, shopping list, and checklists that are printer friendly and stick-on-the-fridge easy to use. Go grab this right now!

· CHAPTER 20 ·

Alkaline Life Fundamental #1: Crowd Out the Bad

This is where we start. Step one is to crowd out the bad. This is the genuine "easy button" to put living alkaline on autopilot to get you amazing results while giving up nothing!

To get straight to the point, right now what I want you to do is forget about giving anything up. While you are getting started, I want you to completely relax about giving up the acid-forming foods, the treats, the vices, the naughty stuff. Just forget about it. If you want it, you can have it.

I promise, this is *not too good to be true.*

This is my Crowd Out the Bad method, and I've taught it to thousands of very happy folks in the Alkaline Life Club over many years.

The simple yet powerful concept is this: *When you are starting out, focus **only** on getting the good food in. Again, focus **only** on putting the **good in**—don't worry about cutting the **bad out**.*

Sound simple?

Good. It should. Because on top of that, there are just three simple rules to follow.

RULE #1: DON'T WORRY ABOUT CUTTING *ANYTHING* OUT

Do what you want. If you still want to have a coffee, have one. If you still want to have meat with your dinner, go for it. If you still want a dessert, have it.

The very slight but powerful distinction here is that you're having a conversation with your subconscious mind and your conscious mind to make considered decisions. You're not mindlessly having these foods; you're consciously allowing yourself the possibility of having them—you're *not* restricting yourself, going cold turkey with anything, or telling your brain that stuff is banned.

Of course, you *could* take this to the extreme and have 10 Mars bars for breakfast, but I trust that you're at least a little bit interested in health, so you'll probably be like most people who come to me—generally pretty healthy, even if just a little bit, but with a few (or many) vices and foods and treats you love (coffee, chocolate, sugar, alcohol, and so on).

But even if you're in the deep-fried-Mars-bar-with-deep-fried-ice-cream-for-breakfast crowd, this will *still* work—it will just take a little longer.

RULE #2: FOCUS ON GETTING THE *GOOD* STUFF *IN*!

So here's the other side of the bargain. You're allowed to completely forget about eliminating the bad stuff, *but* you have to get the good stuff in, and in abundance. You have to eat your greens, you have to have salads, you have to have juices and smoothies, and you have to have healthy fats and veggies. This is the deal.

To make this more real, here are a couple of examples:

- You can still have a steak, *but* you have to have it with a gigantic salad or some steamed veggies topped with omega-3-rich, healthy dressings.
- You can still have a pizza, *but* you have to have loads of veggies on top and serve it with a huge salad.

- You can still have a dessert, *but* your main course needs to have at least 5 servings of veggies with it.
- You can still have a coffee, *but* you have to have at least 300 ml / 10 oz of alkaline water before and, ideally, after.
- You can still have a sneaky treat for a snack, *but* only after you've had some veggies to snack on first, or some nuts and seeds.

The basic (but very effective) premise here is that the good will crowd out the bad, bit by bit. And when you do this, you won't miss the "bad" stuff at all. At base, you do need a lot of the good. This is the mini compromise you have to make to get tons of the good stuff in. When you add in lots of the nutrient-dense, alkaline foods, you'll feel nourished and satisfied. This is your aim. In no way should your diet be full of deprivation *or* low in nutrients. What you do need to do is feel satisfied and full, and if you follow this rule, you'll also feel so much more energized.

To demonstrate what I mean, have you ever eaten takeout or other junk food and felt full at the time, but then find yourself hungry within 45 minutes? These foods are chemically designed to create this *exact* reaction. They are so nutrient poor that your body will tell you that you're hungry, because it works the bulk of the food through your digestive system quickly, and when it receives no nutrients, it asks for more.

This is why people who are on an overly acid-forming diet overeat. Their body is always starved of nutrients and always demands more and more and more of these nutrient-poor but sugar-, gluten-, chemical-, trans fat-, or yeast-rich foods. And the compounding effect is that the more sugar and gluten we eat, the bigger the candida overgrowth in our digestive system gets. And the bigger it gets, the more yeast it craves. This is just one of a dozen vicious cycles that keeps on compounding.

Healthy, alkaline foods, on the other hand, are nutrient dense. When you eat them, you feel satisfied for longer, because they give your body the nutrients it craves. So when you focus on getting the good in, it literally crowds out the bad.

For example, most people would think a salad is not filling. But if you ate a bowl of spinach, arugula, lettuce, tomato, avocado, and quinoa dressed with healthy fats, you'd feel satiated for hours.

This is how focusing on getting the good stuff in works. Each meal, start with whatever you want to eat first, but the plate *must* be clean of the good stuff by the time you finish.

RULE #3: FOLLOW YOUR INSTINCTS

This rule is the best bit. It's what I love so much about this approach. The traditional approach to the alkaline diet (and any healthy-living plan) requires you to start off by cutting out lots of unhealthy stuff and replacing it with healthy stuff. It immediately puts you at a disadvantage and makes it a challenge that you have to battle from day one. When you use the Alkaline Life approach, you let your subconscious decide when you're ready to progress.

Here is how it works: the more alkaline you get, the more alkaline you *will* get. It's like the "rich get richer" analogy. It compounds and builds. You can start as slowly as you like with this approach, because the best part is, as you focus on getting the good stuff in, you will *naturally* start to remove the bad stuff.

There's a combination of conscious and subconscious motivation at play.

Conscious: the better you feel, the more likely you will *want* to make the right choice. After a few days and increasingly over a few weeks, you will find yourself *wanting* to say no to certain foods or drinks because you feel fantastic and you don't want to change that. You'll get more picky with your treats and save your cheat meals for social events that matter, rather than a casual, random dessert or bottle of wine for no reason on a Tuesday night.

Subconscious: your subconscious is a fast learner, and it works on rewards. The longer you do this, the better and better you'll start to feel. Your brain will notice that the action equals a positive response in your body, and it will put two and two together very quickly. It will then start to act as a healthy filter for you. You'll stop noticing temptations, and you'll stop being drawn toward them.

Have you ever been in a good, healthy place in your mind at the grocery store, and as you head down the freezer aisle, you are so focused on finding the tofu or healthy section that you don't even see the ice cream section? This is your brain filtering *for* you.

My Crowd Out the Bad approach is fantastic for this. It allows you to cut foods out and make healthier choices on autopilot, with no pain, hard work, anxiety, stress, or willpower needed. You just get gradually more and more alkaline and more and more healthy, energized, and full of vitality.

Eventually you will have incredible energy and vitality. You will still have a social life, room for flexibility and treats, and a strong motivation ingrained within you that will allow you to have treats without falling off the cliff and going backward for months. The more you do it, the better it gets!

Getting to the health of your dreams is a lot easier than you've been led to believe. Abundant health does not have to be hard or full of pain, sacrifice, willpower, and anxiety. When you start with Crowd Out the Bad, you truly are training your brain to make the right decisions on autopilot. You will keep moving forward, reaching your goals and milestones without conscious effort and with plenty of ease.

The Willpower Fallacy

When it comes to your diet and your food decision-making ability, your willpower is unreliable and flawed. Everyone's is, in a way, from the context of today's modern diet full of processed, highly refined, chemically created foods.

Your willpower is broken.

It is not your fault.

Don't rely on it.

Really, don't.

Willpower isn't some part of our character that we either have or don't have. Nobody really has that much more willpower than the next person (it is slightly affected by genetics, but not a lot). We don't need only more willpower to resist addictive substances like coffee, chocolate, sugar, and cigarettes.

Willpower is, quite simply, a function of your brain. It takes care of focus, task performance, and emotions as well as choices and decision-making. And there are two reasons why it cannot be relied upon to help you to stick with your diet or lifestyle choices:

1. The Phenomenon of Decision Fatigue

This now widely accepted concept really only came to the fore in the late '90s,[1] when studies showed that each day, willpower is a finite resource. When you're faced with something requiring self-control, it uses up your supply of willpower.

This is willpower's flaw number one when it comes to your food choices.

2. The Unreliable Fuel of Willpower

This second flaw is effectively a result of the up-and-down glucose levels that the SMD provides. The area of the brain responsible for willpower is the prefrontal cortex, and more specifically the anterior cingulate cortex within it. This area of the brain is fueled by glucose (and using it also depletes glucose in the body!). The more up and down your blood sugar levels, the more erratic your willpower will function.

When you combine these two factors:

a) willpower gets depleted with every decision needing self-control throughout the day

b) willpower is hugely erratic when your blood sugar dips

Is it any wonder that as the day goes on, the likelihood of you crashing and eating foods you know you shouldn't skyrockets?

You Have 15 Strong Minutes per Day

Most people have only about 15 minutes of self-regulatory capacity available at any given time. And remember, willpower isn't only about whether you resist the cookies or not. Any activity requiring focus—from reading to checking e-mail, to writing that assignment, to helping the kids with their homework—these all deplete your willpower reserves.

Our brains were not designed for this modern life we lead. But we can still thrive. We just must adapt our strategies so we're not relying on our outdated willpower hardware to help us navigate our modern food choices.

If we work with what we *can* control, we can effortlessly bypass temptation, be consistent, and continue to nourish our body and thrive.

Nadine's Story

A health crisis led me to search for a diet or lifestyle change and to join the Alkaline Lifestyle. I was living with so many symptoms that I put down to menopause—extreme fatigue, difficulty concentrating and sleeping, irritability, backache, headaches. But most (if not all) of those symptoms were actually due to gluten and dairy intolerances and a fairly poor diet.

I took my time in applying everything and eventually did the cleanse too. And wow, the difference that it made to my overall well-being was remarkable, and noticeable within days.

The alkaline life makes absolute sense. The fact that the recipes are naturally gluten- and dairy-free makes it so easy. The recipes are delicious, and I feel so good eating them. I never felt overwhelmed, and I haven't felt this good in such a long time.

I sleep well and wake up feeling refreshed. I'm far more productive at work. My outlook is far more positive, as I feel so much healthier and energetic. An early-morning walk or gym workout sets me up for the day. And I don't look for excuses not to go out anymore (well, most of the time, at least!).

· CHAPTER 21 ·

Alkaline Life Fundamental #2: The Four Core Actions

Right now, picture yourself at 80 percent of your biggest health goals, whether that's more energy or less weight, getting out of pain, or getting away from a particular health challenge. Picture what 80 percent of the way to that goal would look like and feel like. And now smile, because you're going to get there in a very short period of time and with ease.

When we talk about my 20/80 approach to health, we're talking about how you can get to 80 percent of your health goals by implementing just 20 percent of the actions each day. These are the Four Core Actions (FCAs), and if you start here, master these, and turn them into daily habits, you *will* get to 80 percent or beyond of your biggest, wildest health and energy goals.

It can be easy to wildly underestimate the benefits you can gain by practicing just a small number of positive actions consistently. But these are the actions that, if you consistently apply them, will give you life-changing results.

PICKING THE RIGHT HABITS IS THE TRICK

The quality of your life right now, in every area (health, wealth, relationships, and so on), is a result of your habits. The things you do daily, many times subconsciously, are reflected in the quality of your life and ultimately your happiness.

Both good habits and bad habits shape who we are. Crowd Out the Bad is the most powerful and enjoyable way of gently, subconsciously breaking bad health habits. By focusing on the *good*, we really do naturally start to move away from the bad.

And now as we get into the FCAs, you will build the *good* habits. And I can promise you, good habits are 10 times harder to break than bad habits are. Bad habits can be broken quickly because we know they don't serve us. Good habits are more likely to stick because we know they serve us; *plus*, the positive feedback loop they create becomes unshakable.

FCAs are the foundation you can always come back to. No matter how daunting, challenging, stressful, or complex your life becomes, you will always be able to come back to the Four Core Actions as your foundation. If you ever get lost on your health journey, the FCAs will be there as your center to bring it back to basics.

The best practices of habit building that come from some of the most remarkable behavioral-change experts such as Charles Duhigg, James Clear, BJ Fogg, and Gretchen Rubin have been baked into the FCAs, so I don't want you to overthink the application of them too much. A lot of the thinking has already been done for you!

Simply follow the steps and get the results.

How to Approach the FCAs

I'll say it again: *baby steps.*

Approach these FCAs one at a time. Pick the one that feels easiest for you, master it, and then move on to the next. You don't have to do them all at once. You can take the time you need.

Let's say you pick hydration. Even if you *just* focus on getting properly hydrated, it will be a game-changer. And then if you *just* focus on hydration until you feel, intuitively, like it's an unshakable habit, then and only then do you move on to the next FCA.

Again, do not underestimate the incredible results that can come from just a small number of powerful actions that you practice consistently.

Baby steps.

Of course, if you jump straight into the 14-Day Meal Plan, a lot of the FCAs are covered right away from the nutrients it includes, so that will fast-track your results. But even if you do jump straight in, I still want you to consciously pick one of the FCAs, study it, focus on it, turn it into a habit, and master it. And then move on to the next.

One step at a time, you will be amazed at how quickly these four actions become habits and the difference they make.

Let's get into them now.

FOUR CORE ACTION #1: GO GREEN WITH 5 TO 7 SERVINGS OF GREEN FOODS DAILY

If you do *just* this one action, you will see an incredible benefit to your health and energy. The sheer volume of vitamins, minerals, and nutrients such as magnesium, iron, potassium, omega-3, sulforaphane, chlorophyll, antioxidants, and anti-inflammatories will make an enormous difference to your life.

The SMD contains practically no greens. I estimate that most people living on an SMD barely get one serving of greens a day. It is no wonder we are seeing such a prevalence of sickness and disease, with so many people living fatigued and in pain. You just cannot live a vibrant life without these nutrients.

To many people, getting five servings of greens each day sounds daunting, but I absolutely assure you, it takes very little effort and remarkably little time.

Five Ways You Can Easily Get Those Greens

These five steps are all ideas you can use to get your greens up to 5 to 7 servings per day. Again, you don't need to do all of them. Just try out the ones that most easily integrate into your day and stick with them.

Go Green Action #1: Have a Daily Green Juice or Smoothie (3 to 5 servings of greens per day)

If I had to pick *one thing* that I could magically make the whole world do, it would be to add a green drink—either a juice or a smoothie—to their daily life. *Just this.*

You can practically hit your target of as much as 3 to 5 servings of greens before you've left the house in the morning!

For a green **juice** (made with a juicer), you're talking greens such as:

- Celery
- Cucumber
- Spinach
- Kale
- Lettuce
- Plus nongreens like turmeric, ginger, capsicum (bell pepper), tomatoes, beets, and so on

And for a green *smoothie* (made with a blender), you're talking:

- Avocado
- Cucumber
- Spinach
- Kale
- Lettuce
- Plus nongreens like coconut or almond milk, cacao, nuts, seeds, coconut oil, chia seeds, and so on

You can have either a juice or a smoothie, or both. I strongly recommend adding both to your life, which makes both a blender and a juicer one of the best investments you will ever make in your life.

There is no magic formula to whether it is better to have more smoothies than juices, or vice versa, so just try to mix it up.

FOUNDATIONAL GREEN JUICE AND SMOOTHIE RECIPES

Here are two of my favorite recipes—one for a juice and one for a smoothie. There's a lot of room for modification, but these give you a good place to start.

. . . .

ALKALINE DETOX GREEN JUICE

Ingredients

2 large handfuls baby spinach leaves
2 large handfuls kale (any variety)
Handful parsley leaves and stems
½ bunch of coriander (cilantro)
1 large cucumber
2 sticks celery
1-inch piece fresh ginger
1 medium lemon
Filtered water or coconut water, to taste

Instructions
Simply pass all the ingredients through your juicer and top up with water to get your desired consistency.

. . . .

. . . .

ALL-DAY ENERGY SMOOTHIE

Ingredients

⅓ cup almonds

⅛ cup cashews

½ ripe avocado

2 handfuls spinach

1 cup unsweetened almond milk

1 cup coconut milk

3 teaspoons coconut oil

3 tablespoons coconut or other nondairy yogurt

1 tablespoon sunflower seeds

1 tablespoon chia seeds

3 tablespoons raw cacao powder

1 tablespoon maca powder (optional)

Instructions

Put everything into your high-speed blender and blend until completely smooth!

. . . .

Go Green Action #2: Have a Simple Side Salad with Every Meal (2 to 4 servings of greens per day)

This is one of our fundamental core steps in the first few weeks of my Alkaline Life Club because:

1. it's so easy to do

2. you don't have to change anything else about your meal

3. it gets results quickly!

You're already eating lunch and dinner every day . . . right? You have this habit already in your life. So let's build on it!

This is a great example of Crowd Out the Bad in action. You don't even need to change what you eat or plan to eat for lunch or dinner. You just add a simple side salad to the meal with the rule that *you must finish the salad*!

We're not talking an elaborate pomegranate, goat cheese, and arugula salad with toasted pepitas and garlic croutons. This salad is simply two handfuls of leafy greens, lemon, oil, done. You can be fancier than that if you like, but this is all it takes to check the box.

If you did this at both lunch and dinner, you would add 4 servings of leafy greens to your day. Just like that. Plus, it will help you with FCA #3, which we'll get into in just a minute.

Go Green Action #3: Wilt Greens into Sauces, Curries, and Stews (1 to 2 servings of greens per day)

Leafy greens are magic; they disappear when you add them to warm meals! This is especially true of spinach. Whenever I'm cooking a pasta sauce, curry sauce, or a soup or a stew, I wilt a serving of spinach per person into it without anyone really noticing! It's a great way to sneak it in without any large effort, and it's especially awesome for those family members who might not be so enthused about greens as you are!

Go Green Action #4: Add Shaved Broccoli to Dishes (1 serving per day)

This is another magic trick to get broccoli into meals without anyone really noticing, so it's great for kids. Whenever you make a meal, whether it's a stir-fry, pasta, curry, stew, soup, or salad, simply grab a floret of broccoli by the stalk and shave the head into the meal. The tiny, little bits disappear, you can get a huge amount of broccoli in there before anyone notices, and it doesn't change the flavor profile of the meal.

Go Green Action #5: Blend Greens into Soups and Sauces (1 to 2 servings per day)

This is another fantastic way to sneak in more greens for your unsuspecting family members! Once your soup is cooked and you're ready to blend it smooth, just throw a few handfuls of raw, leafy greens into the blender at the end. That's the beauty of it! Rarely does a soup, pasta sauce, curry, or stew go by without me blending in a heap of leafy greens.

Other Go Green favorites from my Alkaline Life Club members:

- *Green dips, dressings, and sauces.* Enhance these with greens like spinach and herbs like basil, cilantro, and parsley.
- *Rapid stir-fry as a side.* Do a simple stir-fry of broccoli, kale, asparagus, and ginger dressed in tamari (gluten-free soy sauce), lemon, and a sprinkle of sesame seeds.
- *Huge serving of wilted spinach as a side.* Wilt spinach in a little water, drizzle with healthy oil, and top with Himalayan salt.
- *Kale chips.* Cook kale leaves rubbed in coconut oil under a very low heat in the oven for a crispy, green snack!
- *Lettuce instead of wraps or bread.* Replacing gluten-containing wraps with large lettuce leaves is a win-win.
- *Greens added to cooked breakfasts.* Add a load of spinach to scrambled eggs or tofu to increase the nutrient content and/or serve with some asparagus, broccolini, and kale.

Before we move on, don't stress too much about hitting 7 servings *every* day. Some days you might have 3 to 4, and others you might have 8 to 9. As long as you're getting greens consistently, you'll be rocking it.

ALKALINE GREEN SHAKSHUKA

This is a great example of a recipe where I have consciously tried to increase the green content. It's a delicious, cooked breakfast and something I have most weekends. In just this delicious brekkie, there are 2 to 3 servings of greens.

Ingredients

2 tablespoons olive oil

½ medium onion, diced

4 garlic cloves, minced

9 ounces brussels sprouts, shaved or finely sliced

1 cup peas

1 zucchini, grated

1 teaspoon ground cumin

½ teaspoon salt

¼ teaspoon black pepper

2 cups packed baby spinach

¼ cup fresh cilantro, chopped

1 large avocado, sliced, for garnish

Instructions

1. In a large skillet, heat the olive oil over medium heat.

2. Add the onion and garlic and cook until softened, about 3 to 4 minutes.

3. Add the brussels sprouts, peas, grated zucchini, cumin, salt, and pepper. Cook for 5 to 6 minutes, stirring occasionally, until the vegetables are tender.

4. Add the baby spinach to the skillet and cook until wilted, about 1 to 2 minutes.

5. Sprinkle the chopped cilantro over the greens and top with sliced avocado.

6. Serve hot, and enjoy!

FOUR CORE ACTION #2: HYDRATE WITH 100 TO 120 OUNCES OF WATER PER DAY

I cannot emphasize enough how important enough water is. When people first join my coaching in the Alkaline Life Club, we go through an onboarding process where I ask them a bunch of questions about their current health, diet, and their goals. One of my favorite questions to ask is, "What's your hydration like?" It's amazing how often a slightly tail-between-the-legs answer comes back of, "Oh, I know . . . not enough."

So many of us *know* how important proper hydration is, but we simply don't do it. I think it's a strange quirk of us humans that we tend to overlook or undervalue things that are readily available or abundant while overvaluing things that are scarce or difficult to obtain.

Being hydrated is a good example of this. It is easy and it is cheap. And we *know we should be doing it*. You simply have to drink more water. But this simplicity and ease means we undervalue it. Instead, we try the more difficult things. We get excited about a complicated, new gym routine or miracle, expensive diet program but forget the simple step of being hydrated.

With my Alkaline Life Club members, I put it like this: "I am not willing to talk to you about any supplements, exercise, or anything else until your hydration is dialed in."

You *have* to get your hydration sorted. Dehydration has been linked to weight gain and increased obesity risk,[1] poor cognitive health and cognitive performance,[2] cancer,[3] chronic kidney disease,[4] stone formation,[5] cardiovascular disease,[6] and all manner of other conditions.[7]

Or put another way, *you cannot be healthy and dehydrated.*

And it's important to remember, hydration doesn't have to be *only* plain water. Your hydration intake includes your herbal teas, green juices, smoothies, any of your powdered supplements, broths, and so on. When you add these in, it quickly adds up.

But how much is "enough"?

I've found with my clients that on average, "enough" for 90 percent of people is around 3 to 4 liters (100 to 120 ounces) per day—sometimes a little less, sometimes a little more. If you're well above your target weight, then you may need a little more, and if you have a lot of muscle and/or are exercising vigorously, then you will need more too.

The basic equation to work out your individual needs is: **34 ounces (1 liter) of water per 40 lbs (18 kg or 2.85 stone) of body weight**. For example:

76 kg ÷ 18 kg = 4.2 liters (142 ounces)

or

120 lbs ÷ 40 lbs = 3 liters (100 ounces)

At this stage, do not worry about going from where you are now to 100 ounces in one day. Take it gradually, day by day and step-by-step, until you're able to hit your goal.

Why Don't We Drink Enough?

I find that most people have two difficulties when it comes to staying properly hydrated:

1. Remembering to Drink Enough

This is probably the biggest of the challenges when it comes to hydration—and I've been through this too! You get to the end of the day and think, *Not again . . . I forgot to drink any water!*

At this stage, trying to glug down 100 ounces before bed is probably not a smart idea. You can try, but it won't work out too well for you or your bedmate!

If this is you, don't stress. There are lots of tips and ideas to help you build this habit.

2. Bloat and Toilet Frequency

The second concern is physically feeling able to drink that much without needing to go to the toilet every two minutes and feeling bloated. My advice here is to just take it slowly and build up.

Don't try to go from zero to 120 ounces in 24 hours.

Set yourself a target of 50 ounces (1.5 liters) for the rest of this week, then 70 ounces (2 liters) next week, and 100 ounces (3 liters) the next . . .

The more you get used to it, the more your body will be able to use the water you consume. In the beginning, it will feel like the water is going straight to your bladder, but this will quickly change after a few days.

An analogy I like to use is to imagine your body like a dried-up sponge (lovely, I know!). When you first start drinking water, it's like running that dried-up sponge under a faucet. The water just runs straight over it and down the drain. But little by little, the more you run the water over the sponge, the more it begins to absorb, and after no time at all, the sponge can hold an incredible amount of water to do its job.

Your body is just like this. The more hydrated you get, the more your body will hold comfortably. You won't feel bloated at all. And the more hydrated you get, the less frequently you'll need to go to the toilet. This is the sign that your newfound hydration is getting delivered to the cells and supporting your digestive system, assisting your liver and kidneys, and improving your immunity.

Everything will get easier the more you do it, so just ease in, take it a day at a time. If you mess up one day, don't worry about it! Just have a glass of water then and there and get back on with your plan the next day!

How to Build the Hydration Habit

We go into huge depth on how to build your hydration habit with new Alkaline Life Club members, but for now, I want to run you through a couple of the steps we take, using our Alkaline Life Club Habit Framework.

Habit Linking

The concept of habit linking is very powerful. You can apply this to any new habit you want to build, and we use it heavily in the Alkaline Life Club. The concept is: when you have a new habit you want to build, link it to a habit that already exists.

With hydration, you could link having a big glass of water to some of these simple habits you might already have in your daily life:

- Waking up
- Cleaning your teeth
- Before making breakfast, lunch, or dinner
- Getting to work
- While dropping the kids at school or picking them up
- While at your kids' soccer practice (yes, that's almost daily for me)

It's far easier to remember to have a glass of water or cup of herbal tea by linking it to an already existing habit than to try to add a completely new activity or habit to your day. You can pick any daily activity, task, or chore.

This is something we used heavily back in the early 2000s at that beverage company I mentioned earlier to get people to use our new products. I feel like the firm might have used it for slightly more nefarious reasons, but that being said, it works.

I used this myself to quickly get my daily hydration up to 120 ounces, and believe me, I used to be *terrible* at remembering. I was firmly in the "kicking myself at bedtime because I completely forgot" camp.

Here's what my habit linking looked like:

- Upon waking: 12 oz lemon water
- Pre-breakfast: 8 oz turmeric latte or tea
- While making breakfast: 12 oz water
- Green juice: 8 oz
- After cleaning teeth: 12 oz water
- Arrive at work desk: 8 oz herbal tea
- Making lunch: 12 oz water
- Back to desk after lunch/in the afternoon: 2 x 8 oz herbal tea

- While making dinner: 12 oz water
- Cleaning teeth at night: 12 oz water

Total = 112 ounces or 3.4 liters

You can see in there, I linked my desired new habit of hydration to the existing habits of daily life. Before you know it, you won't even be thinking about it anymore; it will happen subconsciously.

Other Tips from Alkaline Life Club Members

- *Carry a big bottle.* This makes sure you always have your water on you to sip. I personally like to have a big 1-liter (34-ounce) bottle at all times, and when I do, I always drink my 4.2 liters! Really simple, but *so* effective. How many times are you sitting at your desk, thirsty as hell, thinking, *When I finish this task, I'll go get water*, and then two hours later, you're still sitting there thirsty?

- *Set a reminder.* You won't have to do this forever, but I recommend you set an hourly reminder on your phone or watch to remind you to have a big gulp or a glass of water every hour. It's amazing how often you suddenly realize it's lunchtime, and you haven't really had anything to drink!

- *Always have water at your desk.* Simply having a bottle at your desk at all times means that when you do remember, you can tuck straight into it, rather than thinking, *Oh yes, water. Now let me just finish this e-mail first.*

- *Use the power of tea.* Herbal teas are alkaline! Mostly. You really only have to avoid green and white tea, and the rest are caffeine-free and alkaline. I find this is a great way to beat the boredom of plain water, and it gives me at least a liter of hydration per day. My favorites are peppermint, rooibos, caffeine-free chai, ginger, and orange. They're delicious hot or cold!

- *Fill it with flavor.* Water is water, and it's pretty dull. That's okay. Try to see hydration as a source of health and energy rather than a source of flavor. However, remember you can add lemon, mint, lime, grapefruit—all manner of fresh stuff to make water more enjoyable. I'm personally loving lime and mint at the moment. Mint grows like nothing else in the garden too, so you can get it in abundance for free (or in a pot if you live in an apartment).

- *Know your outcome and plan your route to success.* Set goals. Write them down. Track your progress. Read your goals aloud day and night. Honestly, being hydrated is *the* most important part of any health goal and will get you a long way toward where you want to be, whether that is weight loss, weight gain, muscle growth, more energy, better digestion, or better skin.

Again, you cannot be dehydrated and reach your true health potential.

Many of my Alkaline Life Club members pick this as their first FCA to focus on, and I wholeheartedly encourage that. The results you will get from it (including almost instant increased energy and alertness) will make taking on your next FCA so much easier.

FOUR CORE ACTION #3: GET ABUNDANT HEALTHY FATS

Okay, I've said it a few times now, and I hope we are all on the same page: fat will not make you fat. You need it, and it's essential for abundant health and vitality!

Healthy fats will do so much for your health, energy, digestion, skin, immunity, liver, kidneys, hormones, and weight. Your body *craves* these healthy fats.

The fats we need to get in abundance are omega-3s and saturated fat (primarily from coconut).

Omega-3: An "Essential" Fatty Acid

Omega-3 is so important to our health that it's categorized as an essential nutrient. Like vitamins C and E, selenium, and zinc, the body absolutely needs omega-3, but it can't synthesize it itself, and it relies on us to consume it. We have to consume omega-3 fats every day at an amount of 3 grams or more, which is equivalent to around 3 tablespoons of oil.

In the Alkaline Life Plan, we get omega-3 daily through foods such as nuts, seeds, flax oil, chia seeds and chia oil, and leafy greens, and some folks, of course, eat oily fish such as salmon too.

It's actually quite easy to get enough omega-3 if you focus a little energy on it. If you're following some of my habits from the other FCAs, you can habit-link extra omega-3 consumption to them. For example, from FCA #1 (Go Green), if you have the simple side salad with every lunch and dinner, you can dress it in an omega-3-rich salad dressing. And if you're following the habit of having a green smoothie each day, you can add nuts, seeds, chia, or coconut oil to it and check the box that way too.

Simply drizzling all of your meals with healthy fats adds a lot more nutrition than you would think, and alone, it can get you a long way toward your daily goal, if not all the way.

The Essential Ratio of Omega-3 to Omega-6

As we touched on in Chapter 4, not all omega oils are created equal. While omega-6 fats are also polyunsaturated and considered essential, their primary use is to support energy production (like many other nutrients), and if there are too many omega-6 fats circulating in the body, they contribute massively to inflammation.

It is very, very easy to get too much volume of omega-6 in our diet. Too easy.

Remember, the ideal ratio of omega-3 to -6 is 2:1, or even better would be 3:1. However, in the SMD, the ratio is often more like 1:20. Yes, that bad. Omega-6 is found in vegetable and seed oils that are used in processed foods, packaged foods, takeout, and convenience foods, and so many people are unwittingly consuming a ton of it and contributing to a flood of inflammation in the diet.

The easiest fix is to swap in omega-3-rich oils such as flax, chia, hemp, and walnut and swap out the canola, safflower, sunflower, corn, soybean, and cottonseed oils, plus margarine, spreads, and the like. And when you can, replace packaged, convenience foods with real foods you prepare yourself.

As they say, *"Just eat real food."*

The Saturated Fat That's Good for You

As we discussed in Chapter 17, the body needs medium-chain triglyceride fats to support the levels of good HDL cholesterol, decrease harmful LDL cholesterol, and support the brain, endocrine system, digestive system, and metabolism.

While getting saturated fats from high-quality animal protein is still fine, studies tend to show better results when the saturated fats are from plant sources such as coconut.[8] We're aiming for around 1 gram per day of saturated fat, which is around a tablespoon. You can easily reach this with coconut oil, as it's both delicious and so stable that you can use it in cooking. I personally add coconut oil to my smoothies, breakfast oats, turmeric lattes, curries, and sauces.

Can I Overdo the Fat?

As with everything in life, it is possible to overconsume something if you really went out of your way to do so, even water. But your body is very efficient at expelling what it doesn't use or need. There's quite a high upper limit to omega-3 and medium-chain triglycerides, so you can't easily overdose on these fats through whole foods.

Supplements

You don't really need to worry about supplementing with saturated fat, because you need a lot less and it's easy to hit your target with diet alone. But because omega-3s are so important, so, *so beneficial*, and are not as intuitively easy to get enough of each day, I highly recommend you take an omega-3 supplement daily.

It's also very useful in keeping that omega-3-to-6 ratio in order too! If we're getting a minimum of 3 grams of omega-3 daily and eating a mostly alkaline-forming diet, it is likely we will be keeping that essential omega-3-to-omega-6 ratio where it needs to be, at around 2:1 or 3:1.

Fats to Include

Omega-3 (from oily fish, fish roe, nuts, seeds, flax, chia, and leafy greens)

Saturated fats (from coconut oil, coconut milk, coconut cream, and coconuts, plus occasional high-quality animal protein)

Fats to Avoid

Excessive omega-6 and -9 (from vegetable oils such as sunflower and canola, as well as from processed foods)

Trans fats, hydrogenated fats, and *most definitely* spreads such as margarine

---

Easy Ways to Get More Fat

- **Dressings on your side salads.** If you're making a side salad to go with every lunch and dinner as per the Go Green action, you may as well dress it with an omega-3-rich dressing! From doing just this one thing, you'll get 2 to 4 servings of greens and 2 of your 3 tablespoons of healthy omega-3 from just one simple step.

- **Chia pots.** So creamy and full of healthy fats that they can be a dessert, chia pots can be so simple (see recipe on page 257). A recipe with 2 tablespoons of chia seeds would give you close to the 3 grams of omega-3 you are looking for as the baseline.

- **Flax, hemp, and chia toppings on hot and cold cereals.** Simply sprinkle flax, chia, or hemp seeds on your morning oats, or add to your cereal (gluten-free, of course).

- **Fat-rich sauces on veggies and salads.** Make delicious, fat-rich sauces like my Alkaline Caesar Dressing (page 269).
- **Snacking nuts.** Walnuts, macadamias, Brazil nuts, pecans, hazelnuts, and a few almonds or cashews in any combination gives you a great hit of healthy fats.
- **Smoothie additions.** A really easy way to get the fats in is to add flax, chia, hemp, and coconut to your smoothie.
- **Oily fish.** Fish is undoubtedly the food source that is richest in omega-3. If you're a big fish fan, then roe is the most potent source of omega-3 phospholipids, which are especially good for cognitive health. Eating fish up to 3 times per week is absolutely permitted on the Alkaline Life Plan.
- **Turmeric lattes.** Adding this delicious drink to your morning routine gives you an opportunity to get coconut oil at the very start of your day.
- **Coconut oil as cooking oil.** Coconut oil is incredibly safe to cook with and remains very stable under exposure to heat.

Remember, eating healthy fats will not make you gain weight. With healthy omega-3s and plant-based saturated fats, your body simply eliminates what it doesn't need.

FOUR CORE ACTION #4: ADD TURMERIC AND GINGER TO YOUR DIET

While all alkaline-forming foods are anti-inflammatory, turmeric and ginger are so powerful that we want to focus on them daily as one of our FCAs. If you have any form of inflammatory-based pain, excess weight, digestive issues, hormonal issues, or fatigue, you will see a huge benefit, very quickly, from adding turmeric and ginger to your daily diet.

The curcumin in turmeric and gingerols in ginger, as we discussed in Chapter 4, are two of the most potent anti-inflammatories on earth. This is one of those actions where *if all you do is this, you will see huge results.* When new students join with the goal of getting out of inflammatory pain, I double down on this as their first FCA target. And if you're in daily chronic pain, removing that pain is pretty life-changing.

We are aiming for approximately 1 to 2 centimeters each of raw turmeric and ginger every day.

You don't have to use a tape measure!

Fresh vs. Dried Turmeric

While fresh is best, it's not always easily available. Rest assured, dried turmeric is a fantastic alternative. It's very common and easy to find, and so I always recommend having some for the times you can't find (or run out of) fresh turmeric.

However, I give one very strong recommendation: buy organic dried herbs and spices.

Nonorganic spices are often treated with chemicals, contain GMOs, and are irradiated.[9] And if you're in the U.S., virtually all conventional spices are fumigated with hazardous chemicals that are banned in Europe.[10]

The irradiation is a concern too. Food irradiation is the process of using radiation to kill bacteria and other contaminants. Irradiation changes the chemical composition of a spice, potentially creating toxic, carcinogenic by-products in the food and increasing our exposure to free radicals while also destroying beneficial compounds like the curcumin compound in the turmeric[11]—which is what we're eating it for!

For substitution, the easy rule of thumb is to use 1 teaspoon of dried turmeric for 1 centimeter of fresh, peeled turmeric.

I had someone on one of our Alkaline Life Club coaching calls the other day ask me how thick the circumference of the turmeric should be if they are getting 1 to 2 centimeters of it per day. It doesn't need to be this precise! This is a great example of getting bogged down in the details. If you get 5 grams of turmeric today and 10 tomorrow, that's fine. If you get 3 grams today and 6 tomorrow, that's fine too! We're just aiming to get these powerful spices in our life every day.

Easy Ways to Get Your Daily Turmeric and Ginger

- **Turmeric-and-ginger lattes and tea.** I have two core recipes for turmeric-and-ginger drinks. One is a creamy latte style (page 254), and one's a refreshing tea (page 254). Warning: they are both absolutely delicious!

- **Sliced into lemon water.** So many of us have lemon water each morning anyway, so just add some turmeric and ginger! I like to use a vegetable peeler to peel off some superthin slices and just drop them in.

- **Grated into salads.** Simply use a cheese grater to add some turmeric and ginger to your salad. Toss it through, and voilà—you have turmeric and ginger in a very subtle way.

- **Grated into stir-fry.** Similarly, you can grate ginger and turmeric into a stir-fry—I recommend doing this once you've finished cooking and turned off the heat. While it's still in the pan, stir through the grated turmeric and ginger. This is also when I like to add fresh herbs to keep them fresh tasting and as nutrient dense as possible.

- **Blended into soups.** Turmeric goes brilliantly into almost *any* soup. It adds a richness and depth without altering the flavor too much. I like to add about 1 centimeter per person per serving and, as before, once the soup is done and blended. Ginger doesn't work as universally with soups, but you can still add it to many.

- **Juiced and smoothie'd.** You can easily add turmeric and ginger to any juice or smoothie. The flavor will be more noticeable in an all-raw juice or smoothie (compared to some of the other foods), so be careful not to overdo it. But the benefits are so amazing that neither a juice nor smoothie goes by in my house now without this treatment.

- **Tossed with roasted veggies.** This is where turmeric powder comes into its own. Turmeric and ginger go great with roasted cauliflower, broccoli, sweet potato, carrots, and beets—practically everything. Just put all your raw, chopped veggies into a bowl, drizzle with coconut oil, and add a teaspoon of powdered turmeric and ginger— get your hands in there and rub it all over! Then roast as normal, and you're set.

- **Stir through rice or cauliflower rice.** You can use either grated or powdered turmeric and ginger, and it's as simple as it sounds! Once you've cooked the rice or pulsed your cauliflower rice, just stir through some turmeric and ginger.

PUTTING THE FCAS INTO ACTION

I have just given you four actions and 32 ideas to put them into practice. You do not have to do them all! The Four Core Actions, together with Crowd Out the Bad, are the main fundamentals that make up the foundation of the Alkaline Life Plan. They are your North Star that you can always come back to when you need to realign and get back to basics.

With both, I want you to take your time and move at a pace that is right for you.

To reiterate, I recommend focusing first on *one* of these actions. Simply pick the *one* that you feel most confident about. Then focus on *just that one thing*, forgetting *everything else*, until that *one thing* is a habit embedded in your life. Once you're achieving your goal daily without having to even think about it, move on to the next FCA.

One thing, one step at a time. Keep it simple.

As we move into the 14-Day Alkaline Life Plan, get ready for your life to change. I truly believe that. These next 14 days will set the stage for dramatic changes in your health, energy, and body. But it's just the start. The habits we build over these two weeks, with the Alkaline Life Fundamentals as the foundation, will put you on the path to reaching your fullest, most incredible health potential with ease.

Anne's Story

I was stuck in a bit of a rut. I was 73 kilograms (161 pounds) and needed to be 63 kilograms (139 pounds). I needed to get balance in my body and mind. I had been gaining around a kilogram per year for the past few years, and it just sat there.

A couple of years earlier, I had been on a scientific expedition to the Simpson Desert, walking 15 kilometers per day in the searing heat, living with nature, watercourses, crawly insects, flies, seeds you can eat, dingoes, wild camels, birds, soaring eagles, and trees with shade (bliss!). It was hard work, and at night, crawling into my sleeping bag, exhausted, to look up and see the amazing night sky was magical. Walking 10 to 15 kilometers a day before setting up camp and tending to the camels would get me into a meditative state. All the worries of the modern world would subside. I found I had a real balance, a clarity, by the end.

The return to the normal world and modern life soon took this peace and clarity away, and I knew I needed to find a way to return to this state and put my health as a priority.

Following the Alkaline Life, I have lost the weight I needed to, and I feel the benefits are only just starting. I feel healthy, energetic, and light and am in such a good space now both physically and mentally. I feel lighter and in sync inside.

I find I don't get stressed. I listen, and if I can't solve the problem or offer advice for someone that's asking, I just wait now and let it wash over me. If the answer is meant to come, it will. I'm not a particularly spiritual person, but this balance I have is because of the food and exercise I'm doing, I'm sure.

I am 70 and don't really go on social media much, but the community is magnificent. I remember all the good advice and encouragement I got as a newbie, and I know I have progressed because I know how to answer the questions now for the new newbies!

· CHAPTER 22 ·

The 14-Day Alkaline Life Plan
Week One: Getting Started

The goal of this 14-day plan is not to be perfect. It is to take you on a journey from wherever you are now to living a 20/80 alkaline life over the course of two weeks in an easy and enjoyable manner. By the end of these 14 days, you will have tried a lot of new things, and there will be some actions and strategies you love and some you discard. But you'll end the two weeks with an armory of simple steps and new habits that will put a lot of your Alkaline Life on autopilot.

The aim is for this to be a lifestyle that you can effortlessly stick to, not an arduous two weeks that you can't wait to see the end of. We want to embed the 20/80 into *your* alkaline life and build habits that keep giving you results for years and years.

THE OVERVIEW

During these two weeks, we will slowly build the habits of the Four Core Actions, and you'll see my "habit tips" scattered throughout.

We'll focus a lot on habit formation and use the very best science around making behavior change as easy and stickable as possible.

Each week there are Four Core Action Goals, and you can pick one, two, three, or four. I generally recommend starting with just one of the FCAs and then adding more as you feel comfortable, but if you want to move forward at a faster pace, this is absolutely fine too. Trust your intuition.

How the Alkaline Life Meal Plans Work

And there's the Alkaline Life Meal Plan for each week too. If you can follow it as it is set out, you will see incredible results. And I've built it to ease you in! You will see that there are quite a few meal-time slots where I say "Your Usual Meal." These "spare" mealtimes are included to give you the break to simply eat whatever you feel like or would normally eat at that time. However, if you want to progress more quickly and have another alkaline meal in that slot instead, then that's awesome too.

There is also flexibility with the meal plan. It is not so prescriptive that I have planned every nutrient in every meal to be consumed at a specifically set time. If there is a recipe you have tried and loved, feel free to repeat it. If there is a specific recipe or ingredient you know you don't love, feel free to swap another for that recipe or ingredient.

And this is important: each of my recipes serves **two**. This is designed to give you some flexibility. You might be following this meal plan with a partner, but if you're not, you get to make twice as much as you need during the 14 days and have a spare serving as a snack or meal later in the day or to keep in the freezer for another time.

Weekly Optional Snacks

Snacks are a huge help. I've learned over the past 20 years that one of the biggest risks to people falling off track is when they get hungry between meals and just need that quick, easy, healthy snack. *Most* snacks are acid forming and unhealthy. So we need to prepare for this.

For each of the two weeks, I give you two make-ahead bulk snacks you can prep on the weekend, plus another two grab-and-go snacks that are quick and easy to pull together from the foods already on your weekly shopping list.

In Week One, I strongly recommend making the bulk snacks ahead of time on Saturday or Sunday. And if you love one of them, repeat it in Week Two, or try another of the week-two recommendations. None of these take a lot of time to make, and they are all equally *delicious*.

And don't forget, your extra serving of each meal (if you are not doing this with a partner) can be used as a snack too, so make sure to store it for later!

Implementing the FCAs

Alongside following the Alkaline Meal Plans, the big-picture plan is for you to hit your Four Core Action (FCA) goals, with the goal getting bigger and closer toward your ideal as we move through the 14 days.

Note that many of the FCAs will kick into autopilot as you follow the Meal Plan, but I want you to decide which of the FCAs you want to focus on and then follow the advice in Chapter 21 to ensure you are fitting this into your daily routine and habits.

I highly recommend starting the plan on a Saturday, so that you have more time and less stress in your morning routine, and then giving yourself the weekend to get used to some of the things you might be doing for the first time! If you start on Saturday, get into the swing of things, and perhaps even get some meal prep done on Sunday, once Monday comes around (as it always does!), you'll hit your stride and will find your new morning routine a lot quicker and easier. Therefore, you should go shopping with your weekly list on a Friday to make sure you start Saturday morning with your delicious alkaline breakfast and drinks and have all of the ingredients ready to go. If you wake up on Day One and *then* have to go shopping before you can start, it's not ideal.

With that being said, let's get into it!

> **Important:** Go to www.thealkalinelifebook.com to download printer-friendly versions of the Alkaline Life Plan Weekly Meal Plans, recipes, itemized shopping lists, and daily checklists for the 14-Day Plan.

WEEK ONE: GETTING STARTED

Week One Four Core Action Goals

- 1 to 2 servings of healthy fats
- 68 ounces (2 liters) of hydration
- 1 serving anti-inflammatories
- 3 to 4 servings of greens

This first week is all about getting started. It's about doing the simple things right. You will make mistakes and possibly slip up from time to time. This is natural and totally fine.

The focus is on crowding out the bad by adding in the good. So it's natural that you might still have a coffee, a glass of wine, maybe a dessert or some cheese. This is totally acceptable. Honestly! The goal here is to focus first only on getting the good stuff in. Don't let yourself get to a place of anxiety, stress, or craving. Remember from Chapter 20, you need to bypass willpower.

But if you ever do feel like you slip up at all this week, don't give yourself a hard time. What I want you to do instead is embrace it and sit with it for a moment. Reflect on *why*—what were the circumstances, and how were you feeling? Was it simply logistical (you were caught out hungry with nothing healthy available), or was it emotional, or something in between? Just give it a little thought for a minute or so, forgive yourself, and work out how it happened and how to prevent it in the future.

Awareness is key.

Whether it's a soda, an ice cream, or a feast, the most important thing—and a mistake I see a lot of people make—is not to let one slipup derail you. It can be easy to throw in the towel and think, *Well, that's that, I may as well give up now,* or, *I've messed up, so I'll give up for the day (or week, or weekend) and start again tomorrow (next week, when I get back from vacation)* . . . and so on.

There is no reason not to simply dust yourself off and start again. Just commit to a healthy meal, drink, or snack right away and keep on going.

By following the 14-Day Meal Plan, you will hit a lot of your FCA targets or get a long way toward them with the greens, fats, and anti-inflammatory foods you need. But this leaves the hydration goal up to you!

When you break it down, like we did on page 201, it's really simple:

- When you wake up, have a big glass of lemon water.
- Then have your turmeric tea or latte and a juice or smoothie.
- Have a glass of water while you're making breakfast, lunch, and dinner.
- Have a glass of water before or after cleaning your teeth.
- Enjoy some cups of herbal tea at work and during the day.

This schedule gets you comfortably over the baseline of 100 ounces per day. If you were to skip a step or two, you'd still be great. If you were to add a supplement like a green powder in a big glass of water, you'd add a little more.

This plan is designed to get you started building an unshakable foundation, to create those FCA habits and the cycle of results, confidence, consistency, and motivation. Remember, this is not a 14-day crash diet that you struggle through, finish, and breathe a sigh of relief after and then go back to your old ways. This is a two-week plan that is gentle, enjoyable, and uplifting, and it is *just the start*. It has been thought through in detail, planned specifically to make it as simple and easy as possible for you while getting you the biggest, brightest results. Trust the process.

And so we move on to your Week One Meal Plan. Remember, where I say "Your Usual Meal," this is a slot where you can relax and simply have what you'd normally have. Don't stress about it. But if you *want* to pick another alkaline recipe, go for it!

I also include lots of times where you'll have the second serving of the recipe either later in the day or the following day to keep things as simple and cost-effective as possible. This means if you're doing the plan alone, make both servings (remember, all recipes serve two). If you are doing this as a couple, you need to double the quantity.

Delicious Green Juice

To borrow from the Alkaline Life Club Habit Framework once more, another tip for turning desired behaviors into habits is to **make actions more attractive.** When it comes to greens, the best bang-for-your-buck way to get plenty of them is to have a daily green juice or smoothie. But I know this is a first for some people—and maybe you're one of them.

For a lot of green juice first-timers, the taste can sometimes be a little, shall we say, *green*. And I totally get that. What I will say is that your taste buds will definitely evolve over time. It won't be long until you're enjoying that green flavor and savoring the subtle sweetness of the beets and carrots too.

But in the meantime, I don't want you to be put off by green juices and smoothies. We need you to enjoy them from Day One. So let's explore some ways to make a green juice as delicious as possible.

- First and foremost, remove the most bitter, or strongly "green"-tasting ingredients. A hack here is to remove the stems of kale (they are super bitter), and go easy on sea vegetables such as kelp.
- You can add carrots, beets, bell peppers, and tomatoes, which are naturally a little sweeter.

- Use herbs that add a kind of sweetness, such as basil, parsley, or—best yet—mint. These all radically change the taste.
- Add a squeeze of lemon or lime at the end.
- Water the juice down with coconut water instead of regular, filtered water.
- Or instead, use nut milk (like almond or coconut).
- Or just water it down more! It will make the taste less intense.

If you can make the juice as attractive as possible, you'll more likely want to have it each day, and before long, it will be a habit.

This habit "hack" to make an action more attractive can be applied to any part of the Alkaline Life (or any other habit you want to form). Just ask yourself, "How can I make this more attractive?" Can you make it more fun, easier, or more delicious? Can you do it in a fun or enjoyable environment? Give this some thought to take quite a powerful step forward.

WEEK ONE MEAL PLAN

Day One: Saturday

It's Day One! Hopefully life allowed you the time to go shopping last night, and you have woken up excited and ready to go. As you will see, each day in the plan, we wake up and immediately have our delicious, warm, alkalizing, metabolism-stirring lemon water and follow it up with a powerfully anti-inflammatory Turmeric & Ginger Tea or Latte.

I rotate these drinks during the plan, but you can stick with either one or the other or mix it up based on what you prefer that day.

The order of having your alkaline breakfast and your juice or smoothie is totally up to you too. Some days I enjoy the juice while making my breakfast. Other days I'll make the juice or smoothie and pack it to take with me for a midmorning snack.

This first week, you'll note that the morning juice or smoothie repeats in the afternoon for simplicity. Again, you can simply have the second serving later; double the recipe if you're doing it with a partner (though you might have to go shopping again).

The dinner slot today is a "usual" meal, so have whatever you like. If you want to make an alkaline recipe, awesome. If you want to have pizza, awesome. There's zero pressure.

Saturday's Meal Plan

- Before Breakfast: Lemon Water followed by Turmeric & Ginger Tea
- Breakfast: Simple Chai Alkaline Breakfast Oats
- Morning Juice/Smoothie: First serving of Gut Hormone Balance Juice
- Lunch: Hug in a Bowl Lentil Soup
- Afternoon Juice/Smoothie: Second serving of Gut Hormone Balance Juice
- Dinner: Your Usual Meal (you can pick anything!)

Day Two: Sunday

Today you're building on what you've already achieved. You might even be feeling clearer, lighter, and more energized already. By the end of Day Two, it's even more likely, simply from the sheer volume of nourishment your body is now receiving.

Today we are staying with 80 percent alkaline meals, with the dinner slot again being your usual meal. This is by design. The weekend of your first week is often characterized by fantastic motivation and energy during the day and then a bit of a lull in the evening, so we accommodate that.

Today's juice is the Sugar-Craving Busting Smoothie, which can help support you as you hit Day Two. A lot of people really feel the lower sugar in the previous 24 hours today, and this juice has the perfect combination of minerals and fats for killing sugar cravings and balancing blood sugars.

Today might also be a good opportunity to make some of those optional alkaline snacks for the week listed on pages 226 and 227. And this evening, you might also choose to make your juices for tomorrow to save you a little time in the morning.

Storing and Pre-Preparing Juices and Smoothies

Fresh is always best. However, I would rather you add in a few little hacks and shortcuts and stick to the plan instead of aiming for perfection and giving up. Done is better than perfect.

With juices and smoothies, I find they keep quite well for 24 to 36 hours if stored in an airtight container and kept chilled. Light, heat, and air are the enemies of nutrients, and with juices, the taste and texture too. Nobody wants a questionable juice.

So this means you can make your juice or smoothie the night before to save you time in the morning. Or when you make twice the amount you need, you can save your second serving for the next day, effectively cutting your prep time by 50 percent.

Sunday's Meal Plan

- Before Breakfast: Lemon Water followed by Turmeric & Ginger Latte
- Breakfast: Creamy Coconut Chia Pots
- Morning Juice/Smoothie: First serving of Sugar-Craving Busting Smoothie
- Lunch: Second serving of soup from yesterday
- Afternoon Juice/Smoothie: Second serving of Sugar-Craving Busting Smoothie
- Dinner: Your Usual Meal

Day Three: Monday

I go quite light on the amount of preparation work today. This is, for most people, their first day at work on the plan, and so it's best not to overload your morning with complex meals to make for the day ahead.

If you *do* want to take on more, then definitely feel free to have a more alkaline breakfast, and you can even repeat the chia pots from yesterday or make the Chai Alkaline Breakfast Oats.

Lunch could be a simple salad, but you can relax here and just do what you would normally do for your work lunch. And then dinner is my famous 10-Minute Alkaline Dhal. Now, Parmi Mandra, one of my longest-serving students in the Alkaline Life Club, *insists* you cannot truly make a dhal in 10 minutes, but this recipe tastes delicious and takes 10 minutes. That's good enough for me!*

Monday's Meal Plan

- Before Breakfast: Lemon Water followed by Turmeric & Ginger Tea
- Breakfast: Your Usual Meal
- Morning Juice/Smoothie: Brain-Boosting Alkaline Juice
- Lunch: Your Usual Meal
- Afternoon Juice/Smoothie: Second serving of Brain-Boosting Alkaline Juice
- Dinner: 10-Minute Alkaline Dhal

Note: prepare the Chocolate Overnight Oats tonight!

Day Four: Tuesday

You're well into the swing of the working week now and finding that balance with your life. Beginning your day with the hydration of the powerful anti-inflammatory tea or latte and its healthy fats to boost your energy and kick-start your metabolism, alongside

---

* At this stage, Parmi and I agreed to disagree. I concede it's probably not a proper dhal, but we do both agree it tastes good. Brilliantly she just would not dare serve it to her family and say it's a dhal. I'm at peace with that. We're still friends.

the nourishment from your juice and smoothie . . . wow. What a way to start the day!

Today you're having the second serving of the delicious dhal for lunch, so you can quickly pack it to take with you. And to make life even easier, you prepared your breakfast last night too! Your morning is a breeze, and lunch is taken care of. Again, while you can have one of the other delicious alkaline dinner recipes tonight if you like (I personally love the Raw Pad Thai), you can also opt for any regular dish to keep it as easy and stress-free as possible.

Tuesday's Meal Plan

- Before Breakfast: Lemon Water followed by Turmeric & Ginger Latte
- Breakfast: Chocolate Overnight Oats
- Morning Juice/Smoothie: Antioxidant Green Smoothie
- Lunch: Second serving of 10-Minute Alkaline Dhal
- Afternoon Juice/Smoothie: Second serving of Antioxidant Green Smoothie
- Dinner: Your Usual Meal

Day Five: Wednesday

You are now over halfway into Week One, and you're flying! Today the Usual Meal is your work lunch to keep that simple.

With the Alkaline Keto Alfredo Pasta, you'll find that the "pasta" is spiralized zucchini. However, if you want to make it simpler, you can use gluten-free pasta (look for a brand with as few ingredients as possible).

You can spiralize zucchini (known as *courgette* in the U.K.) into noodles using a spiralizer machine. There are other ways of doing it if you don't have (or don't want to buy) a machine. Simply look on YouTube for "how to make zucchini noodles," and you'll see lots of ideas.

Wednesday's Meal Plan

- Before Breakfast: Lemon Water followed by Turmeric & Ginger Tea
- Breakfast: Simple Coconut Chia Pots
- Morning Juice/Smoothie: First serving of Digestive Cleansing Juice
- Lunch: Your Usual Meal
- Afternoon Juice/Smoothie: Second serving of Digestive Cleansing Juice
- Dinner: Alkaline Keto Alfredo Pasta

Day Six: Thursday

Wow, you are nearly at the end of week one already! The ingredients in today's recipes are focused primarily on helping stabilize blood sugar and continuing to tame the inflammation. By this stage of the week, you are already incorporating so many extra healthy fats, greens, anti-inflammatories, and alkaline minerals, and you're likely starting to see how easy it is.

While breakfast has been reserved for a "usual meal," why not experiment with some of the "go green" suggestions in the Four Core Actions and see if you can adapt your usual breakfast by sneaking an extra serve of greens in.

Thursday's Meal Plan

- Before Breakfast: Lemon Water followed by Turmeric & Ginger Latte
- Breakfast: Your Usual Meal
- Morning Juice/Smoothie: First serving of pH-Boosting Alkaline Protein Shake
- Lunch: Second serving of Alkaline Keto Alfredo
- Afternoon Juice/Smoothie: Second serving of pH-Boosting Alkaline Protein Shake
- Dinner: Hug in a Bowl Lentil Soup

Day Seven: Friday

This is the last day of Week One! It's time to celebrate! I've left your Friday night meal as your celebration dinner, so feel free to indulge in whatever you like! If that's takeout or a dinner out with friends or family, that's a great thing to do. Feel free to see it as a "cheat" meal. And if you do, here's what I want you to consider (and honestly, there is no judgment here): think about how good you feel before the meal physically and mentally. Then in the morning when you wake up, absolutely 100 percent commit to getting back onto the plan with your lemon water.

While you're having your lemon water on Saturday, reflect on your energy, mood, health, and feelings inside your body. How has the cheat meal impacted your body and energy? Sit in that feeling for a moment. Then move on.

Cheat meals, date nights, holiday blowouts, a bottle of red when needed—all have a psychological benefit if they're enjoyed in the context of a bigger picture or positive plan. There is a place for them. But as you're starting out, it is useful to have this little conscious reflection on what they give you and what they take away.

Friday's Meal Plan

- Before Breakfast: Lemon Water followed by Turmeric & Ginger Tea
- Breakfast: Simple Alkaline Oats
- Morning Juice/Smoothie: First serving of High-Energy Juice
- Lunch: Second serving of Hug in a Bowl Lentil Soup
- Afternoon Juice/Smoothie: Second serving of High-Energy Juice
- Dinner: Celebration dinner of your choice!

WEEK ONE SNACK OPTIONS

. . . .

COCONUT ENERGY BALLS

Makes approximately 8 to 10 balls

Ingredients

¼ cup cold-pressed coconut oil, room temperature

¼ cup rice malt syrup (brown rice syrup)

⅓ cup cacao or pure cocoa powder

A pinch of sea salt

1 cup raw pecans or walnuts, soaked and dehydrated

⅔ cup shredded, unsweetened coconut

Instructions

1. Cover a dinner plate or small tray with wax paper and set aside.

2. In a medium bowl, combine the coconut oil, rice malt syrup, and cacao powder. Stir and press the mixture until it is thoroughly blended.

3. Stir in the remaining ingredients.

4. With your hands, form ¾-inch round balls and place them on the prepared plate.

5. Freeze the balls for 15 minutes to set.

6. Enjoy cold or thawed.

. . . .

TURMERIC-ROASTED CHICKPEAS

Makes approximately 4 to 6 servings

Ingredients

One-half 15.5-ounce can chickpeas, drained and rinsed

1 tablespoon avocado oil

Pinch of Himalayan salt

1/2 teaspoon turmeric powder

Instructions

1. Preheat oven to 350°F (176°C). Set out a small bare baking sheet.

2. Lay out paper towels (or a clean kitchen towel) and spread the chickpeas out on them. Gently roll and pat the chickpeas dry.

3. In a small bowl, mix all the ingredients.

4. Place the mixture on the baking sheet and bake for approximately 45 to 50 minutes.

CHIA-SEED ENERGY CRACKERS

Makes 12 crackers

Ingredients

1/2 cup chia seeds

1/2 cup sesame seeds

1/2 cup pumpkin seeds

1/2 cup sunflower seeds

1 clove crushed garlic

1/2 teaspoon cayenne pepper

Salt and pepper to taste

1 1/4 cups of water

Instructions

1. Preheat oven to 300°F. Line a baking sheet with parchment paper.

2. Mix together all the ingredients and let sit for 10 minutes for the chia seeds to soak up the water.

3. Using a spatula, spread the mixture onto the baking sheet.

4. Divide the mixture into 12 sections. Bake for 30 minutes.

5. Remove the pan from the oven, flip the crackers over, and bake for another 25 minutes.

6. Once golden and crackable, you know the recipe is ready. Enjoy plain or with optional avocado, or serve with a dip, like hummus.

WEEK ONE SHOPPING LIST

*Asterisks indicate items that will be purchased in excess amounts that can be used during Week Two or in the future.

Fresh Produce

- ❏ 1 apple
- ❏ 2 avocados
- ❏ 1 bunch basil
- ❏ 1 bunch beets with their greens
- ❏ One 6-ounce container blueberries
- ❏ 1 head broccoli
- ❏ 2 heads cabbage (napa or savoy)
- ❏ 8 carrots
- ❏ 1 head cauliflower
- ❏ 2 bunches celery
- ❏ 1 bunch chard
- ❏ One 8-ounce container cherry tomatoes
- ❏ 1 bunch cilantro
- ❏ 6 cucumbers
- ❏ 2 heads garlic
- ❏ About 12 pieces of fresh ginger root (22 inches)
- ❏ 2 bunches kale (about 10 ounces)
- ❏ 9 lemons
- ❏ 1 lime
- ❏ 1 onion
- ❏ 1 bunch oregano
- ❏ 1 bunch parsley
- ❏ One 8-ounce bag fresh or frozen peas
- ❏ 2 red chilies
- ❏ 3 bunches scallions
- ❏ 6 bunches spinach (about 30 ounces)
- ❏ About 10 pieces fresh turmeric root (9 inches)
- ❏ 2 zucchini

Pantry

- ❏ One 16-ounce bag almonds*
- ❏ 32 ounces unsweetened almond milk
- ❏ One 8-ounce bag cacao nibs*
- ❏ One 8-ounce bag cacao powder*
- ❏ One 16-ounce bag cashews*
- ❏ One 16-ounce bag chia seeds*
- ❏ One 15.5-ounce can chickpeas
- ❏ One 15-ounce can coconut cream
- ❏ Four 15-ounce cans coconut milk
- ❏ 32 ounces coconut water
- ❏ One 14-ounce jar coconut oil*
- ❏ 16 ounces coconut yogurt
- ❏ One 8-ounce bag flaxseeds or flax meal*
- ❏ Three 15-ounce cans green lentils

- ❑ One 16-ounce bag oats
- ❑ One 16-ounce bottle olive oil*
- ❑ One 8-ounce bag pine nuts*
- ❑ One 16-ounce bottle rice malt syrup*
- ❑ One box rooibos tea bags*
- ❑ One 2-ounce jar sesame seeds

- ❑ One 8-ounce bottle tamari*
- ❑ Two 32-ounce containers MSG-free, yeast-free vegetable broth
- ❑ One 8-cube box MSG-free, yeast free vegetable bouillon*
- ❑ One 8-ounce bag walnuts*

Spices

- ❑ One 2-ounce jar black pepper
- ❑ One 2-ounce jar ground cinnamon*
- ❑ One 2-ounce jar curry powder*

- ❑ One 2-ounce jar nutmeg*
- ❑ One 4-ounce jar sea salt*
- ❑ One 2-ounce jar cloves*
- ❑ One 2-ounce jar vanilla beans or 1 4-ounce bottle vanilla extract*

Optional

- ❑ Assorted nuts and seeds
- ❑ Two 6-ounce containers assorted berries

- ❑ 16 ounces brown rice, wild rice, or quinoa*
- ❑ One 12-ounce bag shredded coconut*

A Note about Keto and Alkaline

You'll have seen a few recipes pop up with *keto* in the title. The Alkaline Life and keto can be quite easily combined. They are incredibly similar with the focus on healthy fats, almost no sugar, lots of green vegetables, and a lower level of carbs. The only real difference is that with keto, you would be ramping up your fat even more to be closer to 70 to 80 percent of your total calories and keeping carbs at under 10 percent.

Living alkaline can still include more carb-rich foods such as sweet potato, zucchini, and peas, whereas to get into ketosis, you would be limiting these.

If you do want to integrate living alkaline into a keto approach, we have a full program on this inside the Alkaline Life Club, which you can check out at www.thealkalinelifebook.com.

If you want to follow an alkaline-modified keto approach, you can follow most of these recipes, but be sure to increase your fat intake. It is worth noting that some studies are showing that adding more alkaline-forming foods to a ketogenic diet can reduce risk of adverse effects and increase efficacy. This study from 2017 on children following a ketogenic diet found that adding alkaline supplements and food was a great help. They called it "an acidosis-sparing ketogenic diet."[1]

· CHAPTER 23 ·

The 14-Day Alkaline Life Plan
Week Two: Making It Stick

Now that we are into days 8 to 14, you will really start seeing the magic happen. After the first seven days, you will feel phenomenal. In Week Two we build on that, celebrate the wins, recognize the new habits you're forming, and really make this stick.

I encourage you to take some time out to recognize all the wins you've had and consider their impact—not just toward your health goals but in other areas of your life too (what the extra energy and positivity has meant for your relationships, career, hobbies, and so on).

In Week Two, we increase the hydration, fats, greens, and anti-inflammatory foods. You'll see in the meal plan that there are fewer Usual Meals as we increase our intake of those nourishing alkaline-forming foods. On Saturday and Sunday, you'll eat a completely alkaline diet, and then you'll ease off again on Monday. I want you to experience what it's like to go fully alkaline for a few days while you have the time and space at home, away from work and other distractions, so you can get a feel for how great this is for your body, your energy, and your vitality.

We continue with the daily juices and smoothies. Feel free to swap ingredients in and out, or indeed whole recipes, for your daily juice or smoothie. Some will appeal more than others, and that's totally natural.

For the turmeric tea or latte choice, I leave this up to you to decide. Pick which you prefer.

And the hydration should continue to build. Use the habit linking to continue building on the good work you've done in Week One and aim for that goal of 100 to 120 ounces.

WEEK TWO FOUR CORE ACTION GOALS

- 2 to 3 servings of healthy fats
- 100 ounces (3 liters) of hydration
- 2 to 3 servings anti-inflammatories
- 5 to 7 servings of greens

WEEK TWO MEAL PLAN

Day Eight: Saturday

- Before Breakfast: Lemon Water followed by your choice of Turmeric & Ginger Latte or Turmeric & Ginger Tea
- Breakfast: Scrambled Keto Breakfast Brekkie
- Morning Juice: Kidney-Rejuvenation Juice
- Lunch: Tuscan Bean Soup
- Afternoon Smoothie: All-Day Energy Smoothie
- Dinner: Raw Pad Thai

Day Nine: Sunday

- Before Breakfast: Lemon Water followed by your choice of Turmeric & Ginger Latte or Turmeric & Ginger Tea
- Breakfast: Alkaline Green Shakshuka
- Morning Juice: Zesty Lemon & Ginger Green Juice
- Lunch: Crunchy Anti-Inflammation Salad
- Afternoon Smoothie: Digestive-Support Smoothie
- Dinner: Alkaline Detox Curry

Note: Make your Chocolate Overnight Oats tonight to have it ready for Monday, and if time permits, make the Coconut & Buckwheat Noodle Soup so it's ready for lunch at work.

Day Ten: Monday

- Before Breakfast: Lemon Water followed by your choice of Turmeric & Ginger Latte or Turmeric & Ginger Tea
- Breakfast: Chocolate Overnight Oats
- Morning Juice: Digestion Green Juice
- Lunch: Coconut & Buckwheat Noodle Soup
- Afternoon Smoothie: Digestion Green Smoothie
- Dinner: Alkaline Keto Alfredo "Pasta"

Day Eleven: Tuesday

- Before Breakfast: Lemon Water followed by your choice of Turmeric & Ginger Latte or Turmeric & Ginger Tea
- Breakfast: N'Oatmeal
- Morning Juice: Immune-Boosting Juice
- Lunch: Leftover Keto Alfredo Pasta
- Afternoon Smoothie: Keto-Alkaline Green Smoothie
- Dinner: Mexican Stuffed Sweet Potato & Chunky Avo Salsa

Day Twelve: Wednesday

- Before Breakfast: Lemon Water followed by your choice of Turmeric & Ginger Latte or Turmeric & Ginger Tea
- Breakfast: Hidden Greens Oats
- Morning Juice: Triple-A Juice
- Lunch: Shredded Carrot Antioxidant-Boost Salad
- Afternoon Smoothie: Alkaline Detox Smoothie
- Dinner: Creamy "Crunchy" Broccoli Soup

Day Thirteen: Thursday

- Before Breakfast: Lemon Water followed by your choice of Turmeric & Ginger Latte or Turmeric & Ginger Tea
- Breakfast: Alkaline Berry Parfait
- Morning Juice: Immune-Boosting Juice
- Lunch: Leftover Broccoli Soup
- Afternoon Smoothie: Digestive-Support Smoothie
- Dinner: Green Detox Casserole

Day Fourteen: Friday

- Before Breakfast: Lemon Water followed by your choice of Turmeric & Ginger Latte or Turmeric & Ginger Tea
- Breakfast: Turmeric Chai-Spiced Smoothie Bowl
- Morning Juice: Immune-Boosting Juice
- Lunch: Leftover Detox Casserole
- Afternoon Smoothie: Digestive-Support Smoothie
- Dinner: Happy Hormone Vegetable Soup

WEEK TWO MAKE-AHEAD SNACK OPTIONS

. . . .

NO-BAKE BREAKFAST BARS

Makes 8 bars

Ingredients

1 cup coconut cream

2 tablespoons coconut oil

3 tablespoons rice malt syrup (brown rice syrup)

1⅓ cups almond butter

1 inch ginger, grated (or 2 teaspoons ground ginger)

5 cups uncooked oatmeal (quick oats)

Optional: Swap in 1 cup flax meal for 1 cup of oatmeal

Instructions

1. Line an 8 inch x 8 inch baking dish with parchment paper.

2. In a large mixing bowl, whisk the coconut cream, coconut oil, and rice malt syrup until well combined.

3. Add the almond butter and ginger and whisk until combined.

4. Add the oats and mix with a spoon to smooth the mixture all out. If it's still lumpy, you can use your hands to mix it together.

5. Flatten the mixture into the lined baking dish.

6. Refrigerate for a minimum of 2 hours, or overnight, and then cut into bars. These will stay good for at least a week in the fridge.

. . . .

MEXICAN MINI CHOCOLATE CUBES

Makes 12 to 14 mini cubes

Ingredients

½ cup cacao powder

½ teaspoon chili powder

¼ teaspoon cinnamon

⅛ teaspoon nutmeg

1 pinch black pepper

1 pinch fine sea salt

¼ cups cacao butter or coconut butter

¼ teaspoon vanilla extract

25 drops liquid stevia

(Recipe continues)

Instructions

1. Lightly grease 2 mini loaf pans.
2. In a small mixing bowl, mix the cacao powder, chili, cinnamon, nutmeg, pepper, and salt.
3. Melt the cacao butter in a double boiler (a ceramic or glass dish put over a small saucepan of simmering water) until melted.
4. Add the butter, vanilla, and stevia into the dry ingredients and stir until smooth.
5. Divide between the 2 mini loaf pans and allow the mixture to set at room temperature until firm. Then cut it into cubes of the size you would like and store them in an airtight container at room temperature for up to a week.

. . . .

ANTI-INFLAMMATION BLISS BALLS

Makes 8–10 balls

Ingredients

1½ cups almond meal or almond flour

1½ cups shredded, unsweetened coconut

2 teaspoons ground turmeric

1 teaspoon cinnamon

1 teaspoon ground ginger

Pinch of chili powder

½ cup coconut oil

⅓ cup rice malt syrup (brown rice syrup)

Instructions

1. In a medium bowl, combine the almond meal, coconut, turmeric, cinnamon, ginger, and chili powder.
2. Melt the coconut oil over low heat and add the rice malt syrup.
3. Add liquids to the dry ingredients and mix well.
4. Roll the balls into the desired size and refrigerate for 30 minutes.

. . . .

WEEK TWO SHOPPING LIST

*Asterisks indicate items that will be purchased in excess amounts that can be used in the future.

Fresh Produce

- ❏ 8 avocados
- ❏ 3 bunches basil
- ❏ 4 ounces bean sprouts
- ❏ 2 beets
- ❏ 5 bell peppers (red)
- ❏ Two 6-ounce containers blueberries (or other berries)
- ❏ 2 heads broccoli
- ❏ 9 ounces brussels sprouts
- ❏ 1 head cabbage (green or savoy)
- ❏ 2 heads cabbage (red)
- ❏ 17 carrots
- ❏ 4 heads cauliflower
- ❏ Two 12-ounce containers cherry tomatoes
- ❏ 4 bunches cilantro
- ❏ 5 cucumbers
- ❏ 2 sprigs dill
- ❏ 4 heads garlic
- ❏ About 6 pieces of fresh ginger root (11½ inches)
- ❏ 1 jalapeño
- ❏ 10 bunches kale (about 50 ounces)
- ❏ 1 leek
- ❏ 6 lemons
- ❏ 1 head lettuce (little gem or mâche)
- ❏ 3 limes
- ❏ 1 bunch mint
- ❏ 5 onions (yellow)
- ❏ 1 onion (red)
- ❏ 1 bunch oregano
- ❏ 1 bunch parsley
- ❏ Four 8-ounce bags frozen peas
- ❏ 1 potato
- ❏ 1 red chili
- ❏ 16 bunches spinach (about 80 ounces)
- ❏ 1 bunch thyme
- ❏ 1 tomato
- ❏ About 8 pieces fresh turmeric root (9½ inches)
- ❏ 8 zucchini

Pantry

- ❏ One 16-ounce bag almond flour or meal*
- ❏ Two 12-ounce jars almond butter*
- ❏ 32 ounces unsweetened almond milk
- ❏ One 15-ounce can black beans
- ❏ One 8-ounce bag brown rice
- ❏ 32 ounces buckwheat noodles
- ❏ One box caffeine-free chai-spiced tea*
- ❏ One 15.5-ounce can cannellini beans

- ❏ One 15-ounce can coconut cream
- ❏ Three 15.5-ounce cans coconut milk
- ❏ 16 ounces coconut water
- ❏ 16 ounces coconut yogurt
- ❏ One 12-ounce bag shredded coconut*
- ❏ One 8-ounce bag dried cranberries*
- ❏ One 8-ounce jar Dijon mustard*
- ❏ One 4-ounce bag hemp seeds or hearts

- ❏ Two 16-ounce bags oats*
- ❏ One 5-ounce bottle sesame oil*
- ❏ One 8-ounce bag sunflower seeds*
- ❏ One 16-ounce jar tahini*
- ❏ One 10-ounce package tofu
- ❏ One 28-ounce can chopped tomatoes
- ❏ Five 32-ounce containers MSG-free, yeast-free vegetable broth

Spices

- ❏ One 2-ounce jar cardamom*
- ❏ One 2-ounce jar coriander*
- ❏ One 2-ounce jar cumin*

- ❏ One 2-ounce jar garam masala*
- ❏ One 2-ounce jar ground turmeric*

Optional

- ❏ Alkaline sprouted protein powder
- ❏ One bunch Swiss chard

- ❏ Maca powder
- ❏ One 16-ounce bag quinoa or other gluten-free grains

You can download printer-friendly versions of the meal plans, shopping lists, and recipes at www.thealkalinelifebook.com.

· CHAPTER 24 ·

Real-World Living

While we've covered hydration, food, supplements, and the other big-picture elements of living alkaline, there are a few extra day-to-day things you might encounter in your new Alkaline Life.

We want to make this as real-world and achievable as possible, and these factors might be a big help to you.

SLEEP

Most people don't give sleep the credit it deserves. It's essential to get *the best sleep you can*. Being a parent of three young boys, I totally understand how hard this can be at times, and I also roll my eyes at those sleep "experts" who have no kids.

But if you think it will be hard to support your sleep because of your lifestyle (kids, work, pets, shift work, and so on), then you need it now more than ever!

I heard someone explain the importance of sleep on a podcast a few years ago, and while I cannot remember the source (I think even the person who said it couldn't remember the source either!), it really hit home how essential sleep is and how seriously we should take it.

I am paraphrasing, but the suggestion was along the lines of: Think about how we've evolved. Our dominant motivation is survival, and back in prehistoric, paleolithic, or caveman times (whatever you want to call it), our evolution deemed sleep to be *so essential* that it effectively puts us at risk of being eaten by a lion or attacked by a rival, unable to procreate or hunt for a *third* of every day. We are asleep for 8 hours out of 24, unable to strive toward any of our evolutionary targets. And totally at risk. That's how important it is.

It makes sense that we should prioritize sleep. Thankfully there has been somewhat of a global shift away from "I'll sleep when I'm dead" and "hustle, hustle 24/7" that characterized the '80s, '90s, and '00s. And from this, a lot of research and publicity around the importance of sleep and how to get enough good-quality sleep has become much more mainstream.

In the Alkaline Life Club, I see sleep as so important that I am considering making it the fifth Core Action (but it doesn't rhyme, so I might leave it as it is! Kidding!).

20/80 ACTIONS FOR OPTIMIZING SLEEP

- Upon waking, get some exposure to daylight as quickly as possible and for at least 5 minutes. This is a vital trigger for your melatonin/cortisol relationship and cycles.

- Avoid screen time for 30 minutes upon waking. The dull light from your phone, laptop, or tablet is enough to trigger a tiny release of cortisol, but it's so small it doesn't trigger the corresponding hormones that properly manage your sleep-wake rhythm.

- Avoid caffeine for 30 minutes after waking, for the same reason. Give your body the chance to properly, naturally produce the cortisol and adrenaline it needs without spiking it artificially. Also avoid caffeine within 8 hours of bedtime.

- Move your body as close to waking as possible. Combine this with getting the sunlight. Jumping rope, rebounding, or walking are great options.

- Supplements can *really* help. I strongly recommend 145 mg of magnesium threonate, 1,000 milligrams of eicosapentaenoic acid (EPA, one of the two fatty acids in omega-3), and 100 milligrams of theanine, an amino acid. These three will make a big difference. There are many more, but this is the 20/80 of sleep supplements.

- Try to sleep and wake at roughly the same time each day. I know this can be hard, but it does make a massive difference.

These suggestions will help increase the quality of your sleep, and the *quality* of your sleep is as important as the quantity. Try to prioritize this.

EATING OUT

While I always say you should make room and space in your diet for cheat meals, date nights, and guilt-free dinners with friends, there will be times when you eat out more frequently, and you might not want to stray off track with every single meal.

When eating out, you have to accept that some things are out of your control, such as a venue's choice of oils and how it stores them; the ingredients, such as how much sugar or additives it uses in a particular sauce; what's organic or not, and so on.

While I encourage you to be super charming and make requests that you think are doable, you can also apply some simple rules to make the meal as alkaline tweaked as possible.

Rule #1: Pre-Eat!

Simply have an alkaline meal before you go out, ideally within an hour or two of when you'll be eating (not arriving, but actually eating). The best bet here is to aim for a recipe that is high in fat, protein, and fiber. This is the trifecta of satiation. When you hit all three of these, it will keep you satisfied for hours. Note, you don't have to turn up feeling stuffed. You just have to turn up not really hungry!

Rule #2: Juice before You Go

You don't need to have a literal juice; it can be anything that really forwards your progression to your health goal. You could have a smoothie, go for a run, meditate, do some yoga—anything that is a progression to your goal where you might then think, *You know what, I don't want to undo that. I want to keep going.*

I find exercise works best for this. If you have a great workout, you go into your evening with no chance of you wanting to undo the hard work.

If you have a juice, this will also help fill any little nutrient gaps that your brain might interpret as hunger (nutrient deficiency often results in hunger signals).

Rule #3: Superhydrate

Thirst is often also misinterpreted as hunger by your brain,[1] so it's essential you hydrate really well before you go and also continue to while you're at the restaurant. Hunger signals are also easily misinterpreted as low-blood-sugar signals, leading you to the sweet stuff on the menu. You can avoid this trap very easily by simply hydrating. Your goal overall is to have 100 to 120 ounces (3 to 4 liters) each day, so just make sure you're hitting this target!

Rule #4: Research the Menu before You Go

This is now so easy, since practically every restaurant on earth has their menu online these days, whether they want to or not! If you plan out your meal before you go, yes, you lose some excitement for the night, but you can also have far more resolve to make the healthy choices when you get there—regardless of how you're feeling or the specials or what your dining companions order. Temptation disappears.

This also plays nicely with Rule #5 . . .

Rule #5: Ask for What You Want

You can do this at the restaurant *or* before. Please don't be afraid to call beforehand and talk to the restaurant about your needs. If there's literally nothing you can see on the menu that will work for you, just call before, be lovely and polite, and explain your situation—99 times out of 100, the restaurant will want to accommodate you and make the evening special for you.

When you are at the restaurant, be super lovely to your waitstaff, and they'll do everything they can for you (it makes a change from the other grumpy diners they've had that day). I find most chefs love a challenge and the opportunity to do something bespoke (if they have the time!). If the restaurant is super busy, be aware of that and try to make requests as minimal as possible. This is where calling beforehand can really help. If you love the look of entree X but there is no main that works with you, ask if they can combine X into a huge salad. If you love the look of the roasted vegetables that come with main Z, ask if you can combine that with entree Y. You get the gist. Just don't be afraid to ask.

Rule #6: Skip the Bread

This should go without saying. Bread is gluten. It is as acid forming as it gets. Instead of having the bread, see if they have anything in the appetizers you'd enjoy just as much or more, such as olives or another antipasto.

Rule #7: Double Starter

There's a double benefit to the double starter. First, studies show that people are more likely to overeat when they're served bigger portions.[2] If you're going to a restaurant where you know the portions are huge, try ordering two appetizers instead of a main course. This can help you fill up without going overboard, both in terms of the size of the meal and the implicit volume of acid-forming ingredients.

Appetizers are often much more healthy than mains too. They tend to be more simple and fresh. So having two of these instead of one large main can be a far better choice.

Rule #8: Soup for Starters

If you are going to skip Rule #7 above, I recommend ordering a soup to start with. Studies looking at the effects of eating soup before a meal have shown that it can reduce your total food intake by 20 percent, again helping prevent overeating.[3] Even if you decide to have a blowout and order whatever you like (which is totally fine from time to time), it's really important not to overeat as well and put too much stress on your digestive system and liver all at the same time.

Rule #9: Go Slow, Be Mindful

Eat slowly—so slowly that it seems silly. Be mindful while you're eating and stay present to the conversation, the event, and the connection with your dining partners. Make the event about that connection instead of what you're eating. Chew slowly.

The slower you go, the less harmful impact any acid-forming foods will have on your body, especially your digestive system and liver.

Chewing your food thoroughly and eating more slowly can help you eat less.[4] It can also make you feel full more quickly.

Putting your utensils down between mouthfuls is also a good way to slow down and give your brain a chance to recognize when you're full.

Following even two to three of these steps can make a huge difference.

STAYING ALKALINE WHILE TRAVELING

When we are away from home, it is harder to stay alkaline. There is no doubt about that. We don't have access to our usual pantry, juicer, blender, water filter, supplements, healthy lunch spots, fridge, freezer, and so on. You're a lot more reliant on eating out and the small number of things you can pack for your trip.

My big goal for you if you are away from home, whether it's travel for work or fun, is to *double down on those Four Core Actions*!

Don't set your goals too lofty. As they say, *it is what it is*. You can do only so much while you're away from your home, so focus on the FCAs and make them as simple as possible.

Daily Greens

The baseline here is to take a green powder supplement with you so you get your greens each day, guaranteed. On top of this, in a lot of reasonably sized towns and cities, you will be able to find a juice and smoothie shop. Don't buy these bottled in the grocery store, as they'll almost certainly be useless nutritionwise and expensive.

When eating out, remember to order a side salad and a side of green vegetables, which most restaurants have.

And if you can fit it in your luggage, take a mini blender like a small Nutribullet, and you can get all of the ingredients for a basic green smoothie at the grocery store (or have them delivered).

Anti-Inflammatories

The baseline here, too, is your curcumin supplement. Many cafés now sell turmeric lattes, but if you can bring that mini blender, you can also make a simple turmeric-and-ginger latte in your hotel room. If you can't pack a blender, you can still bring powdered turmeric to make a turmeric tea, simply with hot water and a little rice malt syrup or stevia for sweetness.

Hydration

While it is as easy to get your 100-ounce minimum of water when you're away as it is at home, the quality of water is trickier. My pro tip here is to get an alkaline water jug (my recommended equipment is at www.thealkalinelifebook.com) and pack this in your suitcase or even your backpack. I have done this for years. It takes up almost no room in your luggage, as you can simply stuff it full of clothes!

Hydration is so important, so when you're traveling, this really is not only an easy one to keep up with, but it's vitally important too. Don't skip it!

Healthy Fats

Again, the baseline is your supplement, but it's also easy to add extra fats by hitting your other FCA-while-traveling goals. Making your green smoothie? Add avocado, flaxseed, and coconut oil.

Making your turmeric latte? Add coconut oil. Having a salad at a restaurant? Make sure they bring you extra olive oil.

Just keep on adding that fat.

Pack Snacks Too!

When you're heading away, be sure to pack lots of alkaline snacks with you. My favorites are frozen Anti-Inflammation Bliss Balls (page 236), lots of nuts and seeds, my own homemade granola or muesli, and raw chia seeds that I can mix with a can of coconut milk or cream for a quick, delicious breakfast or dessert.

WHAT HAPPENS IF I SLIP UP?

We will all have slipups, myself included, and it's just a part of life. When this happens, it's so important not to let it get you down, or worse, turn it into something that lasts days, weeks, or even months, when really it should just last a minute. Like we've discussed, we don't want to get into that mindset where we have a slipup and then consign the rest of the day, week, or month to the trash can ("Oh well, I've messed up now. I'll start again next week").

When you have a slipup, simply follow these steps:

1. Once you're aware of the slipup, immediately forgive yourself and smile about it. We're all human and flawed, and that's okay.

2. Don't beat yourself up. Think about how much you enjoyed it and have gratitude in the pleasure you got from it.

3. Then let that go. Now switch to the negative outcomes from the slipup. What will it mean, what are the consequences, and what will you now have to do to make up for it?

4. Now get out of emotion and into the analytical part of it. Try to think about what the actual physical steps and logistics were that led you to the slipup. Was there anything you could have done that would have

prevented the opportunity arising? Are there lessons you can take from it?

5. Now, the final step, and this might be a bit woo-woo for some, but close your eyes and try to picture yourself doing the thing you did again, and then make that image as dark and small and dimly lit as possible. Open your eyes. Close your eyes and do it again. Repeat this four or five times. Now close your eyes again and picture yourself taking the action you *wished* you had taken, be it saying no to the cookie or getting water instead of coffee, etc. And now picture yourself doing the right thing and try to embody how that feels. Feel how happy and confident you are, and how proud of yourself you are. Open your eyes. Close your eyes and repeat *this* four or five more times. I *really* urge you to try this. It is a tried-and-tested NLP technique, and it's incredibly powerful.

The most important thing here is, *don't beat yourself up. Forgive yourself, dust yourself off, and move on.*

DAILY PRE-PLANNING

Daily pre-planning is a form of micro goal setting that is such a powerful psychological tool. And it's so simple! All you need to do is this: before you go to bed, write down your plan for tomorrow.

That's it!

Write down roughly what you're going to eat for breakfast, lunch, and dinner. Write down what your hydration will be like and how and when you'll get plenty of water. Make a quick note of any exercise you'll do. Basically you're committing your brain to follow through.

Not only does this microcommitment serve as incredible motivation, but it also creates a plan. When you know what you'll be having for breakfast, you remove the possibility that you'll wake up and be unsure, maybe skip it, or just grab something unhealthy on the way to work.

And you'll be more likely to take the time to make that green juice or pre-prepare your lunch.

And on the flip side, you're far less likely to make *bad* decisions too.

KEEP IT SIMPLE, AND DON'T GET STRESSED!

The last five strategies in this chapter are really just guides for you and for situations and circumstances that might come up. Don't see them as anything other than gentle suggestions from me.

As has been the theme throughout this book, you can get incredible results with just a few of the right actions, practiced consistently.

I am so proud of the fact that if you do only 20 percent of what we have discussed, you will see wonderful changes to your health and energy. And seeing those results, well, maybe it will inspire you to do the next 20 percent, to see even bigger results.

Get started on the 14 Days. Put the simple foundations of Crowd Out the Bad and the Four Core Actions into practice. I promise you, it will deliver you to your true health potential.

· CHAPTER 25 ·

Celebrate!

As you complete the 14-Day Alkaline Life Plan, you are ready to start your own alkaline life. Now is the time to celebrate and reflect on how far you have come. Try to notice every little improvement and benefit you have experienced.

The sheer volume of nourishment you have been giving your body every day is astonishing, certainly compared to the SMD. Just think of how much good your body is doing for itself with the extra vitamins C, E, A, B, and more, plus the extra magnesium, potassium, and iron. Imagine the immune-boosting benefit from the awesome quantities of sulforaphane and your body's increased glutathione levels. Imagine the amount of inflammation that's been tamed from the daily turmeric and ginger; the digestive, cardiovascular, cognitive, and metabolism-boosting impact of the omega-3; the support to your liver and kidneys from the hydration; the endocrine support from the nutrient-rich greens; the bone strengthening from the alkaline minerals; and the blood-building from the chlorophyll.

CREATE A LOVE AFFAIR

I want you to remember that your body loves you. It loves you unconditionally. One of my biggest wishes is that you see yourself and your body as being on the same team. Your body is working constantly to support you by running a myriad of complex, incredibly difficult tasks 24/7/365 to keep you alive. Your blood running through your veins, your lymphatic system pumping, your lungs enabling you to breathe, your glands producing chemicals and hormones, your immune system responding to stimuli (including dealing with those unhealthy foods we eat!), your hypothalamus regulating your temperature, your entire system *regulating your pH* . . .

It does all of this for you. Your only job is to provide your body with the tools it needs. It will do the rest, lovingly, and you will thrive.

Nourishing yourself with real, whole, delicious foods is an incredibly powerful way to reconnect with your body. It is a joy. And it will happen for you.

I cannot wait to hear from you, and where your magical journey takes you. And in my next book, I hope you are one of the success stories I share with the world.

Until then, let's do this!

—Ross

PART IV

Recipes and
Resources

Recipes

Unless stated otherwise, recipes are for two servings. If you're dining solo, consider preparing both servings for leftovers. Also note that in the meal plans, the second serving is often accounted for in either the same day's or the next day's meals.

. . . .

LEMON WATER

Ingredients
2 ½ cups filtered water
½ lemon

Instructions
Warm the water slightly and separate it into 2 glasses. Squeeze the lemon equally into each.

. . . .

. . . .

TURMERIC & GINGER TEA

Ingredients

1 inch fresh turmeric, peeled

1 inch fresh ginger, peeled

2 1/2 cups of filtered water

1/4 lemon

Instructions

1. Grate the turmeric and ginger into a small saucepan, add the water, and bring to a simmer.

2. Simmer for 3 to 5 minutes, and when you're ready to serve, squeeze in the lemon's juice.

3. Serve warm.

. . . .

TURMERIC & GINGER LATTE

Ingredients

1 inch fresh turmeric, peeled

1 1/2 inches fresh ginger, peeled

2 teaspoons coconut oil

1 cup coconut milk

1 teaspoon ground cloves

1 cup coconut water or filtered water

1 vanilla bean or 1/2 teaspoon vanilla extract (optional)

Pinch of black pepper (optional)

Instructions

1. Grate the turmeric and ginger into a mortar.

2. Add the coconut oil. Use the pestle to grind the mixture into a beautiful orange-yellow paste.

3. In a small pan, combine the coconut milk and water, and then add the paste and cloves. If you are using black pepper, you can add it here.

4. Simmer for 4 to 5 minutes.

5. Serve warm, straining if you wish.

. . . .

SIMPLE CHAI ALKALINE BREAKFAST OATS

Ingredients

1 cup rolled oats

2 cups filtered water (preferably alkaline)

1 stick cinnamon (or 1/2 teaspoon ground, plus an additional sprinkle to serve)

1 1/2 teaspoons ground ginger or 1 inch fresh ginger, finely grated

1/2 teaspoon ground nutmeg (preferably fresh)

1 teaspoon ground cloves (optional)

1/2 cup coconut cream or milk, to taste

1 vanilla bean or 1/2 teaspoon vanilla extract

1 apple, if transitioning (optional)

1/2 lemon or lime rind, grated

Sprinkle of assorted seeds and nuts, to taste

1 tablespoon coconut yogurt (optional)

Instructions

1. In a medium-sized bowl, prepare the oats according to the package instructions, using water instead of milk.

2. Stir in the cinnamon, ginger, and nutmeg (and cloves, if using). Add the coconut cream or milk to taste. Scrape out the vanilla bean and add it (or use vanilla extract). Grate in the apple if you're using it.

3. Warm through. To serve, remove the cinnamon stick and add the lemon or lime rind on top and sprinkle with extra ground cinnamon. Top with the seeds and nuts (I recommend sesame seeds with this especially) and coconut yogurt, if using.

GUT HORMONE BALANCE JUICE

Ingredients

1 cup spinach

2 ribs celery

1 medium or large cucumber

1/2 to 1 inch fresh ginger

1 1/2 cups coconut water or filtered water

1/4 lemon

Pinch of ground cinnamon

Instructions

1. Juice everything except the lemon and cinnamon.

2. Stir in the cinnamon, and then squeeze in the lemon.

HUG IN A BOWL LENTIL SOUP

Ingredients

½ tablespoon olive oil

2 carrots, peeled and finely chopped

2 ribs celery, finely chopped

1 onion, finely chopped

2 cloves garlic, grated

1 inch fresh ginger, grated

1 small bunch scallions, finely sliced (plus extra to serve)

4 cups vegetable broth

One 15-ounce can green lentils, drained and rinsed

1 lime, juiced

2 tablespoons tamari

1 red chili, finely chopped plus extra to serve)

Pinch of sea salt

Instructions

1. In a large saucepan over medium heat, heat the olive oil. Add the carrots and celery and cook for 5 minutes until slightly softened. Add the onion, garlic, ginger, and scallions and fry for 30 seconds until fragrant.

2. Pour in the vegetable broth and bring to a boil. Reduce the heat to low and add the green lentils. Simmer for 10 minutes until the vegetables are soft and the soup is slightly reduced. Add the lime juice, tamari sauce, and chili, along with a pinch of salt.

3. Serve hot, with a sprinkle of scallions and chili on top for extra flavor and color.

. . . .

CREAMY COCONUT CHIA POTS

Ingredients

1 cup coconut milk

¼ cup chia seeds

½ teaspoon vanilla extract

1 tablespoon ground flaxseed
or 1 tablespoon flax meal

1 teaspoon sesame seeds

1 cup coconut yogurt

1 teaspoon ground cinnamon,
for garnish

Toppings for 3 varieties:

1 handful blueberries

1 handful mixed nuts (almonds,
macadamia, pistachios,
Brazil nuts, etc.)

1 fig, sliced

Instructions

1. In a large bowl, combine the coconut milk with the chia seeds, vanilla, flax, and sesame seeds.

2. Chill in the fridge for 20 to 30 minutes until the chia has expanded.

3. To serve, fill a small glass with a layer of coconut yogurt, a layer of the chia mix, and then a little extra layer of coconut yogurt.

4. Top with your choice of toppings and sprinkle with cinnamon!

. . . .

SUGAR-CRAVING BUSTING JUICE

Ingredients

1 cup spinach

2 cups kale, stalks removed

¼ head broccoli

¼ cup parsley leaves

1 cucumber

2 ribs celery

Coconut water or filtered water,
to taste

Squeeze of fresh lemon juice
(optional)

Instructions

Juice all the ingredients and top up with coconut water or water to taste. If you want to remove some of the "green" flavor, add a squeeze of lemon juice.

. . . .

BRAIN-BOOSTING ALKALINE JUICE

Ingredients

1 medium cucumber

3 ribs celery

1 handful kale

1 handful spinach

1 small beet

¼ small green cabbage

2 medium carrots

Filtered water or coconut water, to taste

Instructions

Juice all ingredients and add water or coconut water to taste!

10-MINUTE ALKALINE DHAL

Ingredients

1 tablespoon coconut oil

4 cloves garlic, minced

1 inch fresh turmeric, finely chopped

1 inch fresh ginger, finely chopped

5 scallions, roughly chopped

10 cherry tomatoes, halved

½ head broccoli, roughly chopped

1 teaspoon Himalayan salt

One 15-ounce can coconut cream

One-half 15.5-ounce can chickpeas, drained and rinsed

One-half 15-ounce can cooked lentils, drained and rinsed

2 tablespoons curry powder

½ teaspoon black pepper

½ lime, juiced

2 large handfuls spinach

½ bunch cilantro, roughly chopped

Optional to serve: cooked brown rice, wild rice, or quinoa

Instructions

1. In a large pan over medium heat, heat the coconut oil and add the garlic, turmeric, and ginger, stirring for 1 minute.

2. Add the scallions, cherry tomatoes, broccoli, and salt and keep stirring for another 2 minutes.

3. Add the coconut cream (you can add water until you reach your preferred consistency), chickpeas, lentils, spices, and lime juice.

4. Stir in the spinach. Simmer for 2 minutes, until the spinach is wilted. Remove from the heat and top with the cilantro.

5. Serve with rice or quinoa, or simply as a hearty, warming bowl on its own!

. . . .

CHOCOLATE OVERNIGHT OATS

Ingredients

½ cup rolled oats

¾ cup unsweetened almond milk

1 tablespoon rice malt syrup

1½ teaspoons chia seeds

1½ teaspoons cacao powder

1 tablespoon toasted chopped walnuts

1 teaspoon cacao nibs

Instructions

1. In a small bowl or jar, combine oats, milk, syrup, chia seeds, and cacao powder.

2. Cover and refrigerate overnight. Before serving, top with walnuts and cacao.

. . . .

DIGESTIVE CLEANSING JUICE

Ingredients

2 teaspoons chia seeds

A handful of kale

A handful of baby spinach

1 cucumber

2 ribs celery

½ bunch cilantro

½ inch fresh ginger

Coconut water or filtered water to taste

Instructions

Juice all ingredients and add coconut water or water to get the taste and thickness you like.

. . . .

ANTIOXIDANT GREEN SMOOTHIE

Ingredients

1 cup spinach

1 cucumber, chopped

1 avocado

1 inch fresh ginger

1 inch fresh turmeric

1 tablespoon chia seeds

2 tablespoons flaxseed

2 cups brewed rooibos tea, cooled

A few ice cubes

Instructions

1. Blend all ingredients together in a high-speed blender until smooth and creamy. If needed, add filtered water or more rooibos tea to achieve your desired consistency.

2. Serve immediately.

. . . .

ALKALINE KETO ALFREDO PASTA

Ingredients

¼ cup cashews

1 medium head cauliflower, roughly chopped

3 cloves garlic, minced

1 tablespoon avocado oil or coconut oil

2½ cups unsweetened almond milk

1 yeast-free, MSG-free vegetable stock cube

2 teaspoons pine nuts

½ lemon, juiced

½ handful of oregano

½ handful of basil

Himalayan salt and black pepper, to taste

Chili flakes (optional)

1 cup peas, fresh or frozen

2 large handfuls spinach

For the "noodles"

2 carrots, spiralized

2 zucchini, spiralized

Instructions

1. Soak the cashews in warm water so they're easier to blend and set aside.

2. In a medium pan over medium heat, add the cauliflower, garlic, and avocado or coconut oil. Cook for 2 to 3 minutes. Add the almond milk and the stock cube. Bring the mixture to a simmer.

3. Drain the cashews, give them a rinse, and add to the pan. Simmer for 6 to 8 minutes.

4. Pour the pan mixture into a high-speed blender and add the pine nuts, lemon juice, herbs, salt, pepper, and chili flakes (if using). Blend until smooth—and your sauce is ready for the next step.

5. Pour the sauce back into the pan, and over medium heat, add the peas and spinach until they are cooked through. Add the "noodles," heat for 2 minutes, and then serve!

. . . .

PH-BOOSTING ALKALINE PROTEIN SHAKE

Ingredients

1 cup coconut milk

1 cup coconut water

¼ cup filtered water

1 avocado

1 cucumber

1 handful almonds (soaked overnight if you don't have a power blender)

2 handfuls baby spinach

2 scoops sprouted brown rice protein powder

1 tablespoon coconut oil

1 handful chia seeds

1 small handful rolled oats

Instructions

Blend all the ingredients together, starting with the liquids, avocado, cucumber, and spinach. After these, add everything else and blend until smooth.

SIMPLE ALKALINE OATS

Ingredients

1 cup rolled oats

1 cup filtered water

1 tablespoon chia seeds

Coconut or unsweetened almond milk, to taste

1 tablespoon coconut oil

2 teaspoons cinnamon

Coconut yogurt

1 handful mixed nuts/seeds

Berries of your choice (optional)

Instructions

1. In a small pan over medium heat, bring the oats and water to a simmer and then add the chia seeds. Cook until the mixture is a touch too dry for your liking and then stir in a splash or two of the milk (I love coconut milk, but any nondairy milk is fine).

2. Remove from the heat and stir in the coconut oil, cinnamon, and a dollop of the nondairy yogurt. Top with the nuts, seeds, and berries.

. . . .

HIGH-ENERGY JUICE

Ingredients

1 cucumber

2 ribs celery

2 large leaves napa or savoy
   cabbage (or other greens)

3 large chard leaves

2 small beets, including greens

2 large handfuls baby spinach

1 inch fresh ginger

1¼ cups coconut water
   or filtered water

Instructions

Juice all of the ingredients and enjoy!

. . . .

KIDNEY-REJUVENATION JUICE

Ingredients

½ inch fresh turmeric

½ inch fresh ginger

1 red bell pepper

2 handfuls kale

1 cucumber

1 cup coconut water (or to taste)

Instructions

Chop all of the ingredients so that they'll pass through your juicer, and enjoy!

. . . .

SCRAMBLED KETO BREAKFAST

Ingredients

1 tablespoon coconut oil

1 handful kale, roughly chopped

½ yellow onion, chopped

2 tomatoes or 6 cherry tomatoes, diced

10 ounces firm tofu, diced or crumbled

½ small red bell pepper

Pinch of ground turmeric

Freshly ground black pepper

Himalayan or sea salt

Basil, torn, to taste

Instructions

1. In a small pan, add the coconut oil and cook the kale (any variety will do, but I *love* Tuscan kale for this) and onion for 3 minutes.

2. Add the tomatoes, tofu, bell pepper, and turmeric. Add pepper and salt to taste and cook until the tofu is warmed.

3. Top with basil and serve.

TUSCAN BEAN SOUP

Ingredients

2 tablespoons (30ml) olive oil

1 medium onion, chopped

2 ribs celery, chopped

4 cloves garlic, chopped

3 cups chopped tomatoes, with their juice

Three 15.5-ounce cans cannellini beans, drained and rinsed

5 cups filtered water

½ teaspoon Himalayan salt

Freshly ground black pepper, to taste

8 ounces buckwheat pasta, or ½ cup quinoa or other gluten-free grain

2 tablespoons olive oil

¼ cup fresh basil leaves, coarsely chopped

Instructions

1. In a medium pan, heat the olive oil and very gently fry the onions, celery, and garlic until tender over low heat.

2. Add the chopped tomatoes (including their juice) and warm over medium-low heat, breaking up the tomatoes into smaller pieces. Cook for 15 to 20 minutes until everything is infused together.

3. Add the cannellini beans, water, salt, and pepper and cook over medium-low heat for another 20 minutes, until the beans are soft.

4. Add the pasta or grain and cook for another 10 to 15 minutes until al dente.

5. Once the soup has cooled a little bit, stir in the olive oil and add the basil leaves.

. . . .

ALL-DAY ENERGY SMOOTHIE

Ingredients

⅓ cup almonds

⅛ cup cashews

½ ripe avocado

2 handfuls spinach

1 cup unsweetened almond milk

1 cup coconut milk

3 teaspoons coconut oil

3 tablespoons coconut or other nondairy yogurt

1 tablespoon sunflower seeds

1 tablespoon chia seeds

3 tablespoons raw cacao powder

1 tablespoon maca powder (optional)

Instructions

1. Ideally, soak the almonds and cashews overnight. If you're short on time, soaking for a minimum of 20 minutes will suffice.

2. In a blender, combine the avocado, spinach, almond milk, coconut milk, and coconut oil until smooth.

3. Add the almonds, cashews, coconut yogurt, sunflower seeds, and chia seeds. Blend again.

4. Add the raw cacao and, if desired, the maca powder. Keep in mind that maca has a distinct taste, so adjust according to your preference.

5. Once your smoothie is thoroughly mixed, pour it into a glass and enjoy immediately!

. . . .

RAW PAD THAI

Ingredients

3 medium zucchini, spiralized
3 large carrots, spiralized
2 scallions, chopped
1 cup shredded red cabbage
4 ounces bean sprouts
(thoroughly washed)
1 cup cauliflower florets
1 bunch fresh cilantro, roughly
chopped

Sauce
¼ cup tahini
1 teaspoon coconut oil
¼ cup almond butter
¼ cup tamari
Pinch of stevia
2 tablespoons lime or lemon juice
1 clove garlic, minced
1 inch fresh ginger, grated

Instructions

1. In a large bowl, combine the zucchini and carrot noodles, scallions, cabbage, bean sprouts, cauliflower, and cilantro.
2. In a blender, combine all the sauce ingredients. Add a little filtered water if needed—this is a very thick sauce.
3. Mix the sauce into the bowl and get everything evenly coated.

ALKALINE GREEN SHAKSHUKA

Ingredients

2 tablespoons olive oil

½ medium onion, diced

4 cloves garlic, minced

9 ounces brussels sprouts, shaved or finely sliced

1 cup peas

1 zucchini, grated

1 teaspoon ground cumin

½ teaspoon Himalayan or Celtic sea salt

¼ teaspoon black pepper

2 cups packed baby spinach

¼ cup fresh cilantro, chopped

1 large avocado, sliced, for garnish

Instructions

1. In a large skillet, heat the olive oil over medium heat. Add the onion and garlic and cook until softened, about 3 to 4 minutes.

2. Add the brussels sprouts, peas, zucchini, cumin, salt, and pepper. Cook for 5 to 6 minutes, stirring occasionally, until the vegetables are tender.

3. Add the spinach and cook until wilted, about 1 to 2 minutes.

4. Sprinkle the cilantro over the greens and top with sliced avocado.

5. Serve hot and enjoy!

Note: If you are still eating eggs, feel free to add eggs to this dish like a regular shakshuka by creating 3 to 4 "wells" in the mixture while it's in the skillet and cracking in the eggs. Then cover the pan and continue to cook for 5 to 6 minutes.

ZESTY LEMON & GINGER GREEN JUICE

Ingredients

1 cup spinach

1 medium head little gem
    lettuce or mâche

1 rib celery

1 cucumber

½ inch fresh ginger

1 lemon, peeled

Coconut water or filtered water,
    to taste

Instructions

Juice all the ingredients and top up with coconut water or
water to taste.

CRUNCHY ANTI-INFLAMMATION SALAD

Ingredients

5 to 6 cups fresh broccoli florets,
    roughly chopped

¼ cup dried cranberries

¼ cup walnuts, chopped

¼ cup almonds, chopped

½ cup sunflower seeds

1 tablespoon hemp hearts

¼ cup chopped red onion

1 cup frozen peas, thawed

Alkaline Caesar Dressing

1 tablespoon tahini

1 tablespoon Dijon mustard

¼ cup filtered water

1 clove garlic

Himalayan salt and black pepper,
    to taste

Lemon juice, to taste

Instructions

1. In a large bowl, toss to combine the broccoli, cranberries, nuts,
   seeds, onion, and peas.

2. In a food processor or blender, combine all the dressing
   ingredients until smooth.

3. Add the dressing to the salad and toss to mix well; chill
   thoroughly before serving.

ALKALINE DETOX CURRY

Ingredients

Sauce

2 teaspoons coconut oil

½ yellow onion, diced

4 cloves garlic, minced

2 cups steamed sweet potato

1 cup unsweetened almond milk

½ cup filtered water

1 tablespoon curry powder

½ teaspoon garam masala

Pinch of Himalayan salt

Veggies

1 carrot, diced

½ small head of broccoli, roughly chopped

1 zucchini, sliced

1 large sweet potato, sliced

½ cup peas

Rice

½ head cauliflower

Instructions

1. In a medium pan, warm the coconut oil and add the onion and garlic, stirring for around 5 minutes.

2. In a blender, combine the onion-garlic mixture and sweet potato with the remaining sauce ingredients until smooth, and adjust seasoning to taste.

3. Sauté all the veggies until they are tender to your liking, and then pour the curry sauce over them. Turn off the heat, stir through, and let the flavors infuse while you make the cauliflower rice.

4. Break the cauliflower into small chunks and pulse them in a blender until the bits are the size of rice. You can serve this as is or sauté for 1 to 2 minutes in a little coconut oil.

5. Serve the curry atop the cauliflower rice and enjoy!

COCONUT & BUCKWHEAT NOODLE SOUP

Ingredients

1 teaspoon vegetable bouillon powder

One 15.5-ounce can of coconut milk

3⅓ cups boiling filtered water

1 teaspoon sesame oil

½ head cauliflower, cut into small florets

2 tablespoons tamari sauce

2 cloves garlic, minced

10.6 ounces buckwheat noodles

7 ounces broccoli florets, sliced

1 to 2 limes, juiced

6 scallions, thinly sliced, divided

1 handful fresh cilantro, roughly chopped

Himalayan or Celtic sea salt, to taste

1 red chili, thinly sliced (optional)

Instructions

1. In a medium bowl, whisk together the bouillon powder, coconut milk, and boiling water until the bouillon powder dissolves. Set aside.

2. In a large saucepan over medium-high heat, heat the sesame oil. Add the cauliflower and stir-fry for 4 minutes, until slightly softened. Add the tamari sauce and garlic, and stir-fry for another 30 seconds until fragrant.

3. Pour the coconut milk mixture into the saucepan and bring to a boil. Reduce the heat to low, and add the buckwheat noodles and broccoli. Cover the saucepan with a lid and cook according to the noodle package instructions, until the noodles are cooked through and the broccoli is tender but still firm.

4. Add the lime juice, half of the scallions, and cilantro to the soup. Season with salt to taste.

5. Serve the soup hot, garnished with the remaining scallions and sliced red chili (if using).

. . . .

DIGESTIVE SUPPORT SMOOTHIE

Ingredients

½ inch fresh ginger

A handful of baby spinach

A handful of kale, stalks removed

½ bunch cilantro

1 cucumber

1 tablespoon coconut oil

1¼ cup coconut milk

Coconut water, to taste

Instructions

Blend all ingredients and add coconut water to get the taste and thickness you like.

. . . .

KETO-ALKALINE GREEN SMOOTHIE

Ingredients

2 handfuls baby spinach

1 cucumber

4 ribs celery

1 avocado

½ inch fresh ginger

2 tablespoons coconut oil

½ inch fresh turmeric

2 tablespoons chia seeds

1 cup coconut milk

1 cup filtered water

Instructions

Blend all ingredients together and enjoy over ice!

. . . .

IMMUNE-BOOSTING JUICE

Ingredients

1 cucumber

2 ribs celery

1 tomato

1 bell pepper

1 beet

1 handful cilantro

1 cup filtered water (or to taste)

Instructions

Run all of the ingredients through a juicer, running the water through last, and enjoy!

N'OATMEAL

Ingredients

4 tablespoons hemp seeds (hemp hearts)

4 tablespoons almond flour or almond meal

4 tablespoons unsweetened coconut, shredded

2 tablespoons flax meal

2 teaspoons chia seeds

Pinch of Himalayan salt

1 cup filtered water or unsweetened almond milk

Drizzle of rice malt syrup or a pinch of stevia or erythritol (optional)

Dash of vanilla extract (optional)

Instructions

In a small saucepan, add all ingredients and cook for 3 to 5 minutes, adding the syrup, stevia, and/or vanilla at the end.

. . . .

MEXICAN STUFFED SWEET POTATO & CHUNKY AVO SALSA

Ingredients

4 small sweet potatoes

1 tablespoon coconut oil

1 large yellow onion, finely sliced

2 cloves garlic, minced

1 teaspoon ground cumin

1/4 teaspoon ground coriander

One 15-ounce can black beans, rinsed and drained

Salsa

1 cup sweet cherry tomatoes, quartered

1/4 small red onion, diced finely

Olive oil, to taste

1 fresh lime, juiced

Sea salt and black pepper

1 clove garlic, minced

1/2 avocado, chopped chunky

Pea & Mint Guacamole

3 medium avocados, chopped

1/4 cup frozen peas, blanched, minced

1 sprig mint, finely chopped

1 scallion, finely sliced

1 tablespoon fresh lime juice

1 tablespoon jalapenos, minced (optional)

Himalayan sea salt and black pepper, to taste

Olive oil, to taste

Instructions

1. Preheat a convection oven or air fryer to 350°F (180°C).

2. Wrap each potato in foil and place on a baking tray. Bake for around 1 hour, or until each is soft in the middle.

3. While the potatoes are cooking, make the filling. Start by very gently heating the coconut oil in a frying pan. Add the onions and sauté over medium-low heat for 5 to 8 minutes or until onions are soft, and then add garlic. Stir until the onions caramelize.

4. Stir the cumin, coriander, and black beans through the onions and then set aside.

5. In a small bowl, mix the salsa ingredients.

6. In another small bowl, mix the guacamole ingredients.

7. Once the potatoes are cooked through and cool enough to handle, remove the foil and cut lengthwise to create an opening. Spoon filling into each sweet potato and top with salsa and guacamole.

. . . .

HIDDEN GREENS OATS

Ingredients

3/4 cup rolled oats

Pinch of Himalayan salt

1 cup coconut or unsweetened almond milk

1/2 medium zucchini, finely shredded or grated

1/2 cup spinach, finely shredded

1 tablespoon cacao powder

1 scoop alkaline, sprouted protein powder (optional)

1 tablespoon rice malt syrup to sweeten (optional)

1 tablespoon almond butter

Instructions

1. In a saucepan over medium heat, combine the oats, salt, and coconut or almond milk and stir until most of the milk has been absorbed.

2. Stir the zucchini and spinach through the oat mixture until combined, and then add the cacao powder.

3. Reduce the heat and warm through for a further 3 to 4 minutes, and then remove from the heat.

4. If using the protein powder and sweetener, stir these in now and then pour the mixture into your serving bowl. Top with almond butter and serve.

TRIPLE-A JUICE

Ingredients

2 handfuls spinach

2 handfuls kale

1/2 cucumber

1 rib celery

1/2 inch fresh ginger

1/2 inch fresh turmeric

1 red bell pepper

1/2 beet

1 carrot

Filtered water, to taste

Instructions

Juice everything together and enjoy!

SHREDDED CARROT ANTIOXIDANT-BOOST SALAD

Ingredients

6 medium carrots, shredded

¼ red onion, finely sliced

1 red bell pepper, finely sliced

⅛ red cabbage, finely sliced

⅓ cup alkaline Caesar dressing (see Crunchy Anti-Inflammation Salad on page 269 for recipe)

Pinch of Himalayan sea salt

Pinch of black pepper

Instructions

In a salad bowl, stir all of the ingredients until well combined.

ALKALINE DETOX SMOOTHIE

Ingredients

½ avocado

1 cup unsweetened almond or coconut milk

2 large handfuls baby spinach

2 large handfuls kale, stalks removed

¼ bunch fresh cilantro

¼ bunch fresh mint

½ cucumber

1 tablespoon grated fresh ginger

1 tablespoon chia seeds

Instructions

Blend all of the ingredients, starting with the avocado and almond or coconut milk.

GREEN DETOX CASSEROLE

Ingredients

½ cup brown rice

1 tablespoon coconut oil

½ leek, finely chopped

1 rib celery, finely chopped

2 cloves garlic, finely chopped

½ savoy cabbage, finely shredded

1 tablespoon rice malt syrup

½ cup yeast-free, MSG-free vegetable stock

¼ bunch parsley

2 tablespoons fresh dill

Himalayan salt and black pepper, to taste

Instructions

1. Preheat the oven to 350°F (180°C).

2. Cook the rice according to the package instructions and set it aside.

3. While the rice is cooking, in a large pan over medium heat, gently heat the coconut oil. Stir in the leek, celery, and garlic, cooking gently for 3 to 4 minutes.

4. Add the savoy cabbage and rice malt syrup and stir for a further 5 minutes.

5. Transfer cabbage mixture to an ovenproof bowl or large baking dish, and stir in the rice and stock. Bake for 12 to 15 minutes or until most of the liquid is absorbed.

6. Serve in bowls, and top with the parsley and dill. Season with salt and pepper to taste.

CREAMY "CRUNCHY" BROCCOLI SOUP

Ingredients

1 head broccoli

2 tablespoons coconut oil

1 small yellow onion, roughly chopped

3 cloves garlic, crushed

1 small potato, peeled and chopped

5 cups (1.25 L) yeast-free, MSG-free vegetable stock

7 small sprigs thyme, divided

2 tablespoons olive oil

Himalayan or Celtic sea salt, to taste

Black pepper, to taste

2 tablespoons almonds, roughly chopped

1 lemon, juiced, and rind finely grated

1 small handful baby spinach leaves

1 tablespoon Dijon mustard

Instructions

1. Preheat the oven to 440°F (230°C).

2. Cut the broccoli into small florets, reserving about 1/4, and then chop the stems into 1/2-inch pieces and combine with the remaining florets.

3. In a large saucepan over medium heat, gently heat the coconut oil. Add the onion and garlic and cook very gently for 1 to 2 minutes. Add ¼ of the broccoli, plus the potato, stock, and half of the thyme.

4. Bring to a simmer and allow to cook gently for around 20 to 25 minutes or until the potatoes are tender.

5. In a large bowl, combine the remainder of the broccoli, the remaining thyme, and the olive oil. Season with Himalayan salt and pepper, to taste.

6. Spread over a baking tray and bake for 10 minutes, and then toss the almonds through. Bake for another 10 minutes, or until the broccoli is charring. Remove from the oven and sprinkle with the lemon rind. Set aside.

7. Transfer the potato mixture to a blender and add the spinach and mustard. Blend until totally smooth.

8. Now it's time to serve! Divide the soup into bowls and top with the charred broccoli and almonds, and then drizzle with the lemon juice, some extra olive oil, and seasoning to taste.

ALKALINE BERRY PARFAIT

Ingredients

2 tablespoons chia seeds

2 tablespoons filtered water

3 tablespoons unsweetened
shredded coconut

Pinch of ground cinnamon

Pinch of ground cardamom

Pinch of Himalayan salt

2 tablespoons coconut oil

½ cup mixed berries, plus more
for topping (blueberries are
best)

¾ cup coconut cream

¾ cup coconut yogurt

Instructions

1. Preheat the oven to 300°F (150°C). Line a small baking sheet
with parchment paper.

2. Put the chia seeds into a glass with water, stir, and allow them to
thicken and absorb the water.

3. In a small bowl, mix the coconut with the spices and salt, and stir
through the coconut oil. Spread on the prepared baking sheet
and bake for 5 minutes, then remove and allow to cool.

4. In nice, wide glasses, layer the fruit, chia, coconut cream,
coconut mix, and coconut yogurt, finishing ideally with a topping
of the fruit!

. . . .

TURMERIC CHAI-SPICED SMOOTHIE BOWL

Ingredients

16 ounces coconut or
  unsweetened almond milk

2 chai tea bags

1 to 2 teaspoons fresh turmeric,
  grated

Pinch of ground cinnamon

1 tablespoon chia seeds

1 tablespoon rice malt syrup

1 tablespoon almond butter

¼ cup rolled oats

1 scoop plant-based protein
  powder or collagen powder
  (optional)

2 to 3 frozen coconut milk cubes
  (optional, for thickness)

1 handful berries

Coconut flakes, to taste

Instructions

1. In a small saucepan, gently heat the nut milk on the stove. Then
   add the tea bags, turmeric, and cinnamon and gently simmer for
   5 to 6 minutes.

2. Remove the tea bags and then pour the milk mixture into a
   blender along with the chia, syrup, almond butter, oats, and
   protein or collagen (if you're using one of them), and frozen
   coconut cubes, if using. Blend until smooth and pour into a
   large jar.

3. Refrigerate for a minimum of 1 hour to cool and thicken (though
   you can make this the night before and leave it overnight).

4. To serve, divide into 2 bowls and top with a sprinkle of cinnamon,
   berries, coconut flakes, and optionally some chopped nuts.

. . . .

HAPPY HORMONE VEGETABLE SOUP

Ingredients

1 tablespoon coconut oil

½ onion, diced

4 cloves garlic, minced

2 carrots, diced

32 ounces vegetable broth

2 teaspoons Himalayan salt

½ teaspoon ground black pepper

2 teaspoons grated fresh turmeric

6 ounces kelp noodles, roughly chopped

1 bunch chard or kale, thinly sliced, stalks removed

Instructions

1. In a large pot, gently warm the coconut oil and add the onions and a pinch of salt. Sauté the onion for 3 to 4 minutes and then add the garlic and stir for another 30 seconds. Add the carrots and stir well.

2. Add the broth and then salt and pepper to taste, and bring to a simmer for around 15 minutes or until the carrots are al dente.

3. Add the turmeric and kelp noodles and cook for 2 to 3 minutes. Then add the chard or kale, and cook gently until your greens have wilted. Remove from the heat.

4. Add more salt and pepper as needed and serve immediately.

Food Charts

ALKALINE-FORMING FOODS			
Vegetables			
Asparagus	Basil	Beetroot	Broad Beans
Broccoli	Brussels sprouts	Cabbage	Carrot
Cauliflower	Celery	Chard	Chili peppers
Cabbage	Chives	Collards	Coriander/ Cilantro
Cucumber	Dandelion	Eggplant/ Aubergine	Endive
Garlic	Green Beans	Kale	Kelp
Lettuce	Onion	Parsley	Peas
Pepper/Capsicum	Pumpkin	Radish	Runner Beans
Snowpeas	Spinach	String Beans	Sweet Potato
Wakame	Watercress	Zucchini/ Courgette	
Fruit			
Avocado	Coconut	Grapefruit	Lemon
Lime	Tomato		
* Lower sugar berries are the best of the rest, including strawberries, blueberries, and raspberries.			
Nuts and Seeds			
Almonds	Cashews	Chia Seeds	Coconut
Flax Seeds	Hazelnuts	Macadamia nuts	Pumpkin seeds
Sesame seeds	Sunflower seeds		

Sprouts			
Alfalfa sprouts	Amaranth sprouts	Barley grass	Broccoli sprouts
Fenugreek sprouts	Soy sprouts	Wheatgrass	* Any other sprout works!
Breads			
Gluten-/yeast-free breads and wraps	Sprouted bread	Sprouted wraps	
Grains, Beans, and Pulses			
Amaranth	Brown rice	Buckwheat	Lentils
Lima beans	Millet	Mung beans	Navy beans
Pinto beans	Quinoa	Red beans	Soy beans
White beans			
Oils			
Avocado oil	Coconut oil	Flax oil	MCT oils
Olive oil	Pumpkin seed oil		
Spices			
Cardamom	Cinnamon	Cloves	Ginger
Turmeric			
Other			
Alkaline water	Herbal teas	Oily, wild-caught fish (in moderation)	

ACID-FORMING FOODS			
Meat			
Bacon	Beef	Corned beef	Lamb
Organ meats	Pork	Rabbit	Turkey
Veal	Venison		
Seafood			
Clams	Lobster	Oysters	Prawns
Other crustaceans			
Fruits (should be kept to 1–2 servings per day)			
Apple	Apricot	Berries	Cantaloupe
Cranberries	Dried fruit	Grapes	Mango
Melon	Orange	Peach	Pear
Pineapple	Plum	Raspberries	Strawberries
Tropical fruits			
Dairy			
Cheese	Eggs	Ice Cream	Milk
Sour Cream			
Drinks			
Alcohol	Black tea	Carbonated water	Cocoa
Coffee	Colas	Dairy milk	Decaffeinated drinks
Diet drinks	Energy drinks	Flavored water	Fruit juice
Green tea	Sports drinks	Tap water	
Sweeteners and Sugars			
Agave syrup	Any refined sugar	Artificial sweeteners	Carob
Coconut syrup	Corn syrup	Date syrup	Fructose
High fructose corn syrup	Honey	Maple syrup	Molasses
Fats and Oils			
Any cooked oil (except coconut)		Canola	
Other Omega-6-rich vegetable oils		Partially or fully hydrogenated oils	
Safflower	Sunflower	Solid oils (margarine)	

Condiments			
Ketchup	Mayonnaise	Pickles	Soy Sauce
Store-bought sauces	Tabasco	Vinegar	
Other			
Gluten (wheat, spelt, rye, and barley)	Monosodium glutamate	Mushrooms	Vinegars
Natural and Artificial Flavors		Natural and Artificial Colors	

For the full Acid/Alkaline Food Chart go to Resources at www. thealkalinelifebook.com.

Shopping Lists

WEEK ONE SHOPPING LIST

*Asterisks indicate items that will be purchased in excess amounts that can be used during Week Two or in the future.

Fresh Produce

- ❑ 1 apple
- ❑ 2 avocados
- ❑ 1 bunch basil
- ❑ 1 bunch beets with their greens
- ❑ One 6-ounce container blueberries
- ❑ 1 head broccoli
- ❑ 2 heads cabbage (napa or savoy)
- ❑ 8 carrots
- ❑ 1 head cauliflower
- ❑ 2 bunches celery
- ❑ 1 bunch chard
- ❑ One 8-ounce container cherry tomatoes
- ❑ 1 bunch cilantro
- ❑ 6 cucumbers
- ❑ 2 heads garlic

- ❑ About 12 pieces of fresh ginger root (22 inches)
- ❑ 2 bunches kale (about 10 ounces)
- ❑ 9 lemons
- ❑ 1 lime
- ❑ 1 onion
- ❑ 1 bunch oregano
- ❑ 1 bunch parsley
- ❑ One 8-ounce bag fresh or frozen peas
- ❑ 2 red chilies
- ❑ 3 bunches scallions
- ❑ 6 bunches spinach (about 30 ounces)
- ❑ About 10 pieces fresh turmeric root (9 inches)
- ❑ 2 zucchini

Pantry

- ❏ One 16-ounce bag almonds*
- ❏ 32 ounces unsweetened almond milk
- ❏ One 18-ounce bag cacao nibs*
- ❏ One 8-ounce bag cacao powder*
- ❏ One 16-ounce bag cashews*
- ❏ One 16-ounce bag chia seeds*
- ❏ One 15.5-ounce can chickpeas
- ❏ One 15.5-ounce can coconut cream
- ❏ Four 15.5-ounce cans coconut milk
- ❏ 32 ounces coconut water
- ❏ One 14-ounce jar coconut oil*
- ❏ 16 ounces coconut yogurt

- ❏ One 8-ounce bag flaxseeds or flax meal*
- ❏ Three 15-ounce cans green lentils
- ❏ One 16-ounce bag rolled oats
- ❏ One 16-ounce bottle olive oil*
- ❏ One 8-ounce bag pine nuts*
- ❏ One 16-ounce bottle rice malt syrup*
- ❏ 1 box rooibos tea bags*
- ❏ One 2-ounce jar sesame seeds
- ❏ One 8-ounce bottle tamari*
- ❏ Two 32-ounce containers MSG-free, yeast-free vegetable broth
- ❏ One 8-cube box MSG-free, yeast free vegetable bouillon*
- ❏ 1 8-ounce bag walnuts*

Spices

- ❏ One 2-ounce jar black pepper
- ❏ One 2-ounce jar ground cinnamon*
- ❏ One 2-ounce jar curry powder*

- ❏ One 2-ounce jar nutmeg*
- ❏ One 4-ounce jar sea salt
- ❏ One 2-ounce jar cloves*
- ❏ One 2-ounce jar vanilla beans or 1 4-ounce bottle vanilla extract*

Optional

- ❏ Assorted nuts and seeds
- ❏ Two 6-ounce containers assorted berries

- ❏ 16 ounces brown rice, wild rice, or quinoa*
- ❏ One 12-ounce bag shredded coconut*

WEEK TWO SHOPPING LIST

*Asterisks indicate items that will be purchased in excess amounts that can be used in the future.

Fresh Produce

- ❑ 8 avocados
- ❑ 3 bunches basil
- ❑ 4 ounces bean sprouts
- ❑ 2 beets
- ❑ 5 bell peppers (red)
- ❑ Two 6-ounce containers blueberries (or other berries)
- ❑ 2 heads broccoli
- ❑ 9 ounces brussels sprouts
- ❑ 1 head cabbage (green or savoy)
- ❑ 2 heads cabbage (red)
- ❑ 17 carrots
- ❑ 4 heads cauliflower
- ❑ Two 12-ounce containers cherry tomatoes
- ❑ 4 bunches cilantro
- ❑ 5 cucumbers
- ❑ 2 sprigs dill
- ❑ 4 heads garlic
- ❑ About 6 pieces of fresh ginger root (11½ inches)
- ❑ 1 jalapeño

- ❑ 10 bunches kale (about 50 ounces)
- ❑ 1 leek
- ❑ 6 lemons
- ❑ 1 head lettuce (little gem or mâche)
- ❑ 3 limes
- ❑ 1 bunch mint
- ❑ 5 onions (yellow)
- ❑ 1 onion (red)
- ❑ 1 bunch oregano
- ❑ 1 bunch parsley
- ❑ Four 8-ounce bags frozen peas
- ❑ 1 potato
- ❑ 1 red chili
- ❑ 16 bunches spinach (about 80 ounces)
- ❑ 1 bunch thyme
- ❑ 1 tomato
- ❑ About 8 pieces fresh turmeric root (9½ inches)
- ❑ 8 zucchini

Pantry

- ❑ One 16-ounce bag almond flour or meal*
- ❑ Two 12-ounce jars almond butter*
- ❑ 32 ounces unsweetened almond milk

- ❑ One 15-ounce can black beans
- ❑ One 8-ounce bag brown rice
- ❑ 32 ounces buckwheat noodles

- ❏ One box caffeine-free chai-spiced tea*
- ❏ One 15.5-ounce can cannellini beans
- ❏ One 15.5-ounce can coconut cream
- ❏ Three 15.5-ounce cans coconut milk
- ❏ 16 ounces coconut water
- ❏ 16 ounces coconut yogurt
- ❏ One 12-ounce bag shredded coconut*
- ❏ One 8-ounce bag dried cranberries*
- ❏ One 8-ounce jar Dijon mustard*

- ❏ One 4-ounce bag hemp seeds or hearts
- ❏ Two 16-ounce bags rolled oats
- ❏ One 5-ounce bottle sesame oil*
- ❏ One 8-ounce bag sunflower seeds*
- ❏ One 16-ounce jar tahini*
- ❏ One 10-ounce package tofu
- ❏ One 28-ounce can chopped tomatoes
- ❏ Five 32-ounce containers MSG-free, yeast-free vegetable broth

Spices

- ❏ One 2-ounce jar cardamom*
- ❏ One 2-ounce jar coriander*
- ❏ One 2-ounce jar cumin*

- ❏ One 2-ounce jar garam masala*
- ❏ One 2-ounce jar ground turmeric*

Optional

- ❏ Alkaline sprouted protein powder
- ❏ 1 bunch Swiss chard

- ❏ Maca powder
- ❏ One 16-ounce bag quinoa or other gluten-free grains

Go to www.thealkalinelifebook.com to download printer-friendly versions of the Alkaline Life Plan Weekly Meal Plans, recipes, itemized shopping lists, resources, and daily checklists for the 14-Day Plan.

Metric Conversion Chart

Standard Cup	Fine Powder (e.g., flour)	Grain (e.g., rice)	Granular (e.g., sugar)	Liquid Solids (e.g., butter)	Liquid (e.g., milk)
1	140 g	150 g	190 g	200 g	240 ml
¾	105 g	113 g	143 g	150 g	180 ml
⅔	93 g	100 g	125 g	133 g	160 ml
½	70 g	75 g	95 g	100 g	120 ml
⅓	47 g	50 g	63 g	67 g	80 ml
¼	35 g	38 g	48 g	50 g	60 ml
⅛	18 g	19 g	24 g	25 g	30 ml

Useful Equivalents for Cooking/Oven Temperatures			
Process	Fahrenheit	Celsius	Gas Mark
Freeze Water	32° F	0° C	
Room Temperature	68° F	20° C	
Boil Water	212° F	100° C	
Bake	325° F	160° C	3
	350° F	180° C	4
	375° F	190° C	5
	400° F	200° C	6
	425° F	220° C	7
	450° F	230° C	8
Broil			Grill

Useful Equivalents for Liquid Ingredients by Volume				
¼ tsp			1 ml	
½ tsp			2 ml	
1 tsp			5 ml	
3 tsp	1 tbsp		½ fl oz	15 ml
	2 tbsp	⅛ cup	1 fl oz	30 ml
	4 tbsp	¼ cup	2 fl oz	60 ml
	5⅓ tbsp	⅓ cup	3 fl oz	80 ml
	8 tbsp	½ cup	4 fl oz	120 ml
	10⅔ tbsp	⅔ cup	5 fl oz	160 ml
	12 tbsp	¾ cup	6 fl oz	180 ml
	16 tbsp	1 cup	8 fl oz	240 ml
	1 pt	2 cups	16 fl oz	480 ml
	1 qt	4 cups	32 fl oz	960 ml
			33 fl oz	1000 ml	1 L

Useful Equivalents for Dry Ingredients by Weight		
(To convert ounces to grams, multiply the number of ounces by 30.)		
1 oz	1/16 lb	30 g
4 oz	¼ lb	120 g
8 oz	½ lb	240 g
12 oz	¾ lb	360 g
16 oz	1 lb	480 g

Useful Equivalents for Length			
(To convert inches to centimeters, multiply the number of inches by 2.5.)			
1 in			2.5 cm
6 in	½ ft		15 cm
12 in	1 ft		30 cm
36 in	3 ft	1 yd	90 cm
40 in			100 cm	1 m

Endnotes

Chapter 1

1. Park et al., "High Dietary Acid Load Is Associated with Risk of Breast Cancer: Findings from the Sister Study," *The FASEB Journal* 31, no. 51 (2017): 168.4, https://doi.org/10.1096/fasebj.31.1_supplement.168.4.

2. Parohan et al., "Dietary Acid Load and Risk of Hypertension: A Systematic Review and Dose-Response Meta-Analysis of Observational Studies," *Nutrition, Metabolism and Cardiovascular Diseases* 29, no. 7 (2019): 665-75, https://doi.org/10.1016/j.numecd.2019.03.009.

3. Pistollato et al., "Associations between Sleep, Cortisol Regulation, and Diet: Possible Implications for the Risk of Alzheimer Disease," *Advances in Nutrition* 7, no. 4 (2016): 679-89, https://doi.org/10.3945/an.115.011775.

4. Williams et al., "Dietary Acid Load, Metabolic Acidosis and Insulin Resistance—Lessons from Cross-Sectional and Overfeeding Studies in Humans," *Clinical Nutrition* 35, no. 5 (2016): 1084-90, https://doi.org/10.1016/j.clnu.2015.08.002.

5. "The Top 10 Causes of Death," World Health Organization, https://www.who.int/en/news-room/fact-sheets/detail/the-top-10-causes-of-death.

6. Akter et al., "Dietary Acid Load and Mortality among Japanese Men and Women: The Japan Public Health Center-Based Prospective Study," *The American Journal of Clinical Nutrition*, 106, no. 1 (2017): 146-54, https://doi.org/10.3945/ajcn.117.152876.

7. Hejazi et al., "Dietary Acid Load and Mortality from All Causes, CVD and Cancer: Results from the Golestan Cohort Study," *British Journal of Nutrition* 128, no. 2 (2022): 237-43, https://doi.org/10.1017/S0007114521003135.

8. Fereidouni et al., "Diet Quality and Dietary Acid Load in Relation to Cardiovascular Disease Mortality: Results from Fasa PERSIAN Cohort Study." *Food Science and Nutrition* 11, no. 3 (2023): 1563-71, https://doi.org/10.1002/fsn3.3197.

9. Frassetto et al., "Diet, Evolution and Aging: The Pathophysiologic Effects of the Post-Agricultural Inversion of the Potassium-to-Sodium and Base-to-Chloride Ratios in the Human Diet," *European Journal of Nutrition* 40 (2001): 200–13, https://doi.org/10.1007/s394-001-8347-4.

10. I. F. Robey, "Examining the Relationship between Diet-Induced Acidosis and Cancer," *Nutrition and Metabolism (London)* 9, no. 72 (2012), https://doi.org/10.1186/1743-7075-9-72.

11. Park et al., "Association between the Markers of Metabolic Acid Load and Higher All-Cause and Cardiovascular Mortality in a General Population with Preserved Renal Function," *Hypertension Research* 38 (2015): 433–8, https://doi.org/10.1038/hr.2015.23.

12. Williams et al., "Dietary Acid Load, Metabolic Acidosis and Insulin Resistance."

13. Akter et al., "Dietary Acid Load and Mortality among Japanese Men and Women."

Chapter 2

1. Louise McDanell and Frank P. Underhill, "Studies in Carbohydrate Metabolism: XIV. The Influence of Alkali Administration upon Blood Sugar Content in Relation to the Acid-Base-Producing Properties of the Diet," *Journal of Biological Chemistry* 29, no. 2 (1917): 227–32, https://doi.org/10.1016/s0021-9258(18)86786-2.

2. J. A. Tobey, "The Question of Acid and Alkali Forming Foods," *American Journal of Public Health* 26 (1936): 1113–6, https://ajph.aphapublications.org/doi/pdf/10.2105/AJPH.26.11.1113.

3. I should point out that there are many, many fantastic doctors out there too. Many of my students in the Alkaline Life Club found me because their doctor recommended me.

4. Tucker et al., "Potassium, Magnesium, and Fruit and Vegetable Intakes Are Associated with Greater Bone Mineral Density in Elderly Men and Women," *The American Journal of Clinical Nutrition* 69, no. 4 (1999): 727–36, https://doi.org/10.1093/ajcn/69.4.727.

5. König et al., "Effect of a Supplement Rich in Alkaline Minerals on Acid-Base Balance in Humans," *Nutrition Journal* 8, no. 23 (2009), https://doi.org/10.1186/1475-2891-8-23.

6. J. Pizzorno, L. A. Frassetto, and J. Katzinger, "Diet-Induced Acidosis: Is It Real and Clinically Relevant?" *British Journal of Nutrition* 103, no. 8 (2010): 1185–94, https://doi.org/10.1017/S0007114509993047.

7. I. F. Robey, "Examining the Relationship between Diet-Induced Acidosis and Cancer," *Nutrition and Metabolism (London)* 9, no. 72 (2012), https://doi.org/10.1186/1743-7075-9-72.

8. Williams et al., "Dietary Acid Load, Metabolic Acidosis and Insulin Resistance—Lessons from Cross-Sectional and Overfeeding Studies in Humans," *Clinical Nutrition* 35, no. 5 (2016): 1084-90, https://doi .org/10.1016/j.clnu.2015.08.002.

9. V. Rosival, "Dangers of Very Low Blood pH," *Indian Journal of Critical Care Medicine* 15, no. 3 (2011): 194, https://doi.org/10.4103/0972-5229.84887.

10. Pizzorno, Frassetto, and Katzinger, "Diet-Induced Acidosis."

11. K. W. Lee and D. Shin, "Positive Association between Dietary Acid Load and Future Insulin Resistance Risk: Findings from the Korean Genome and Epidemiology Study," *Nutrition Journal* 19, no. 137 (2020), https://doi.org/10.1186/ s12937-020-00653-6.

12. R. S. Williams, P. Kozan, and D. Samocha-Bonet, "The Role of Dietary Acid Load and Mild Metabolic Acidosis in Insulin Resistance in Humans," *Biochimie* 124 (2016): 171-7, https://doi.org/10.1016/j.biochi.2015.09.012.

13. Chan et al., "Higher Estimated Net Endogenous Acid Production May Be Associated with Increased Prevalence of Nonalcoholic Fatty Liver Disease in Chinese Adults in Hong Kong," *PLoS One* (2015), https://doi.org/10.1371/ journal.pone.0122406.

14. C. Passey, "Reducing the Dietary Acid Load: How a More Alkaline Diet Benefits Patients With Chronic Kidney Disease," *Journal of Renal Nutrition* 27, no. 3 (2017): 151-60, https://doi.org/10.1053/j.jrn.2016.11.006.

15. L. Della Guardia, C. Roggi, and H. Cena, "Diet-Induced Acidosis and Alkali Supplementation," *International Journal of Food Sciences and Nutrition* 67, no. 7 (2016): 754-61, https://doi.org/10.1080/09637486.2016.1198889.

16. E. Hopkins, T. Sanvictores, and S. Sharma, "Physiology, Acid Base Balance. [Updated Sep 12, 2022]." In book: *StatPearls* [Internet] (Treasure Island, FL: StatPearls Publishing, 2022), https://www.ncbi.nlm.nih.gov/books/ NBK507807/

17. Frassetto et al., "Acid Balance, Dietary Acid Load, and Bone Effects-A Controversial Subject," *Nutrients* 10, no. 4 (2018): 517, https://doi.org/10.3390/ nu10040517.

18. Buclin et al., "Diet Acids and Alkalis Influence Calcium Retention in Bone," *Osteoporosis International* 12, no. 6 (2001): 493-9, https://doi.org/10.1007/ s001980170095.

19. Sakhaee et al., "Effects of Potassium Alkali and Calcium Supplementation on Bone Turnover in Postmenopausal Women," *The Journal of Clinical Endocrinology & Metabolism* 90, no. 6 (2005): 3528-33, https://doi.org/10.1210/ jc.2004-2451.

20. Buclin et al., "Diet Acids and Alkalis."

21. K. Tucker, M. Hannan, and D. Kiel, "The Acid-Base Hypothesis: Diet and Bone in the Framingham Osteoporosis Study," *European Journal of Nutrition* 40 (2001): 231-7, https://doi.org/10.1007/s394-001-8350-8.

22. Angéloco et al., "Alkaline Diet and Metabolic Acidosis: Practical Approaches to the Nutritional Management of Chronic Kidney Disease," *Journal of Renal Nutrition* 28, no. 3 (2018): 215–20, https://doi.org/10.1053/j.jrn.2017.10.006.

23. Lambert et al., "The Effect of Supplementation with Alkaline Potassium Salts on Bone Metabolism: a Meta-Analysis," *Osteoporosis International* 26 (2015): 1311–8, https://doi.org/10.1007/s00198-014-3006-9.

24. Buclin et al., "Diet Acids and Alkalis."

25. S. A. Lanham-New, "The Balance of Bone Health: Tipping the Scales in Favor of Potassium-Rich, Bicarbonate-Rich Foods," *The Journal of Nutrition* 138, no. 1 (2008): 172S–7S, https://doi.org/10.1093/jn/138.1.172S.

26. Trinchieri et al., "Effect of Potential Renal Acid Load of Foods on Urinary Citrate Excretion in Calcium Renal Stone Formers," *Urological Research* 34, no. 1 (2006): 1–7, https://doi.org/10.1007/s00240-005-0001-9.

27. Ferraro et al., "Dietary Protein and Potassium, Diet-Dependent Net Acid Load, and Risk of Incident Kidney Stones," *Clinical Journal of the American Society of Nephrology* 11, no. 10 (2016): 1834–44, https://doi.org/10.2215/CJN.01520216.

28. Trinchieri et al., "Potential Renal Acid Load and the Risk of Renal Stone Formation in a Case-Control Study," *European Journal of Clinical Nutrition* 67, no. 10 (2013): 1077–80, https://doi.org/10.1038/ejcn.2013.155.

29. Vezzoli et al., "Dietary Style and Acid Load in an Italian Population of Calcium Kidney Stone Formers," *Nutrition, Metabolism and Cardiovascular Diseases* 25, no. 6 (2015): 588–93, https://doi.org/10.1016/j.numecd.2015.03.005.

Chapter 3

1. M. M. Adeva and G. Souto, "Diet-Induced Metabolic Acidosis," *Clinical Nutrition* 30, no. 4 (2011): 416–21, https://doi.org/10.1016/j.clnu.2011.03.008.

2. Carnauba et al., "Diet-Induced Low-Grade Metabolic Acidosis and Clinical Outcomes: A Review," *Nutrients* 9, no. 6 (2017): 538, https://doi.org/10.3390/nu9060538.

3. J. Pizzorno, L. A. Frassetto, and J. Katzinger, "Diet-Induced Acidosis: Is It Real and Clinically Relevant?" *British Journal of Nutrition* 103, no. 8 (2010): 1185–94, https://doi.org/10.1017/S0007114509993047.

4. I. F. Robey, "Examining the Relationship between Diet-Induced Acidosis and Cancer," *Nutrition and Metabolism (London)* 9, no. 72 (2012), https://doi.org/10.1186/1743-7075-9-72.

5. Shi et al., "Dietary Acid Load and the Risk of Pancreatic Cancer: A Prospective Cohort Study," *Cancer Epidemiology, Biomarkers and Prevention* 30, no. 5 (2021): 1009–19, https://doi.org/10.1158/1055-9965.EPI-20-1293.

6. Han et al., "Association between Dietary Acid Load and the Risk of Cardiovascular Disease: Nationwide Surveys (KNHANES 2008-2011)." *Cardiovascular Diabetology* 15, no. 122 (2016), https://doi.org/10.1186/s12933 -016-0436-z.

7. M. Williamson, N. Moustaid-Moussa, and L. Gollahon, "The Molecular Effects of Dietary Acid Load on Metabolic Disease (The Cellular PasaDoble: The Fast-Paced Dance of pH Regulation)," *Frontiers in Molecular Medicine* 1 (2021), https://doi.org/10.3389/fmmed.2021.777088.

8. Akter et al., "Dietary Acid Load and Mortality among Japanese Men and Women: The Japan Public Health Center–Based Prospective Study," *The American Journal of Clinical Nutrition* 106, no. 1 (2017): 146–54, https://doi .org/10.3945/ajcn.117.152876.

9. S. A. Lanham-New, "The Balance of Bone Health: Tipping the Scales in Favor of Potassium-Rich, Bicarbonate-Rich Foods," *The Journal of Nutrition* 138, no. 1 (2008): 172S-7S, https://doi.org/10.1093/jn/138.1.172S.

10. S. A. Lanham-New, "The Balance of Bone Health."

11. Alferink et al., "Diet-Dependent Acid Load—The Missing Link between an Animal Protein–Rich Diet and Nonalcoholic Fatty Liver Disease?" *The Journal of Clinical Endocrinology and Metabolism* 104, no. 12 (2019): 6325-37, https://doi.org/10.1210/jc.2018-02792.

12. Martínez et al., "Extracellular Acidosis Triggers the Maturation of Human Dendritic Cells and the Production of IL-121," *The Journal of Immunology* 179, no. 3 (2007): 1950-9, https://doi.org/10.4049/jimmunol.179.3.1950.

13. Ronco et al., "Dietary Acid Load and Lung Cancer Risk: A Case-Control Study in Men," *Cancer Treatment and Research Communication* 28 (2021): 100382, https://doi.org/10.1016/j.ctarc.2021.100382.

14. Han et al., "Association between Dietary Acid Load."

15. Alferink et al., "Diet-Dependent Acid Load."

16. Robey, "Examining the relationship."

17. Valentina Vicennati et al., "Cross-Talk between Adipose Tissue and the HPA Axis in Obesity and Overt Hypercortisolemic States," *Hormone Molecular Biology and Clinical Investigation* 17, no. 2 (2014): 63-77, https://doi.org/10.1515/ hmbci-2013-0068.

18. Joshua J. Joseph and Sherita H. Golden, "Cortisol Dysregulation: The Bidirectional Link between Stress, Depression, and Type 2 Diabetes Mellitus," *Annals of the New York Academy of Sciences* 1391, no. 1 (2016): 20-34, https://doi.org/10.1111/nyas.13217.

19. Peter E. Stokes, "The Potential Role of Excessive Cortisol Induced by HPA Hyperfunction in the Pathogenesis of Depression," European Neuropsychopharmacology 5 (1995): 77-82, https://doi.org/10.1016/0924-977x(95)00039-r.

20. Michael S. Sagmeister, Lorraine Harper, and Rowan S. Hardy, "Cortisol Excess in Chronic Kidney Disease – a Review of Changes and Impact on Mortality," *Frontiers in Endocrinology* 13 (2023), https://doi.org/10.3389/fendo.2022.1075809.

21. Robey, "Examining the relationship."

22. Williamson, Moustaid-Moussa, and Gollahon, "The Molecular Effects of Dietary Acid Load."

Chapter 4

1. T. Remer and F. Manz, "Potential Renal Acid Load of Foods and its Influence on Urine pH," *Journal of the American Dietetic Association* 95, no. 7 (1995): 791-7, https://doi.org/10.1016/S0002-8223(95)00219-7.

2. Frassetto et al., "Acid Balance, Dietary Acid Load, and Bone Effects-A Controversial Subject," *Nutrients* 10, no. 4 (2018): 517, https://doi.org/10.3390/nu10040517.

3. A study from the U.K. found that sadly, only 8 percent of children and 27 percent of adults get close to this on a daily basis, even though it contains things such as baked beans, canned foods, fruit juice, and ketchup. In the U.K., even a can of Peppa Pig pasta shapes counts. While it has 10 g of sugar per serving, I can guarantee it contains absolutely zero nutrients from vegetables.

4. Belinda Mortell, "Are We Achieving 5-a-Day?" British Dietetic Association, August 13, 2019, https://www.bda.uk.com/resource/are-we-achieving-5-a-day.html#:~:text=Typically%2C%20adults%20eat%20around%20four,5%2DA%2DDDay%20recommendation.

5. J. Di Noia, "Defining Powerhouse Fruits and Vegetables: A Nutrient Density Approach," *Preventing Chronic Disease* 11 (2014): 130390, https://doi.org/10.5888/pcd11.130390.

6. Egner et al., "Chlorophyllin Intervention Reduces Aflatoxin-DNA Adducts in Individuals at High Risk for Liver Cancer," *Proceedings of the National Academy of Sciences of the United States of America* 98, no. 25 (2001): 14601-6, https://doi.org/10.1073/pnas.251536898.

7. Triantafyllidi et al., "Herbal and Plant Therapy in Patients with Inflammatory Bowel Disease," *Annals of Gastroenterology* 28, no. 2 (2015): 210-20, https://www.ncbi.nlm.nih.gov/pmc/articles/PMC4367210/.

8. Tânia Martins et al., "Enhancing Health Benefits through Chlorophylls and Chlorophyll-Rich Agro-Food: A Comprehensive Review," *Molecules* 28, no. 14 (2023): 5344, https://doi.org/10.3390/molecules28145344.

9. Appian Subramoniam et al., "Chlorophyll Revisited: Anti-Inflammatory Activities of Chlorophyll a and Inhibition of Expression of TNF-α Gene by the Same," *Inflammation* 35, no. 3 (2011): 959-66, https://doi.org/10.1007/s10753-011-9399-0.

10. Jiang et al., "Efficacy and Tolerability of an Acne Treatment Regimen with Antiaging Benefits in Adult Women: A Pilot Study," *The Journal of Clinical and Aesthetic Dermatology* 11, no. 6 (2018): 46–51, https://www.ncbi.nlm.nih.gov/pmc/articles/PMC6011872/.

11. S. Nagini, F. Palitti, and A. T. Natarajan, "Chemopreventive Potential of Chlorophyllin: A Review of the Mechanisms of Action and Molecular Targets," *Nutrition and Cancer* 67, no. 2 (2015) 203–11, https://doi.org/10.1080/01635581.2015.990573.

12. P. Thejass and G. Kuttan, "Immunomodulatory Activity of Sulforaphane, a Naturally Occurring Isothiocyanate from Broccoli (*Brassica oleracea*)," *Phytomedicine* 14, no. 7–8 (2007): 538–45, https://doi.org/10.1016/j.phymed.2006.09.013.

13. Kim et al., "Nrf2 Activation by Sulforaphane Restores the Age-Related Decrease of TH1 Immunity: Role of Dendritic Cells," *Journal of Allergy and Clinical Immunology* 121, no. 5 (2008): 1255–61.e7, https://doi.org/10.1016/j.jaci.2008.01.016.

14. R. T. Ruhee and K. Suzuki, "The Integrative Role of Sulforaphane in Preventing Inflammation, Oxidative Stress and Fatigue: A Review of a Potential Protective Phytochemical," *Antioxidants* 9, no. 6 (2020): 521, https://doi.org/10.3390/antiox9060521.

15. J. Kim, "Pre-Clinical Neuroprotective Evidences and Plausible Mechanisms of Sulforaphane in Alzheimer's Disease," *International Journal of Molecular Sciences* 22, no. 6 (2021): 2929, https://doi.org/10.3390/ijms22062929.

16. Yao et al., "Flavonoids in Food and Their Health Benefits," *Plant Foods for Human Nutrition* 59 (2004): 113–22, https://doi.org/10.1007/s11130-004-0049-7.

17. A. Y. Chen and Y. C. Chen, "A Review of the Dietary Flavonoid, Kaempferol on Human Health and Cancer Chemoprevention," *Food Chemistry* 138, no. 4 (2013): 2099–107, https://doi.org/10.1016/j.foodchem.2012.11.139.

18. Melim et al., "The Role of Glucosinolates from Cruciferous Vegetables (Brassicaceae) in Gastrointestinal Cancers: From Prevention to Therapeutics," *Pharmaceutics* 14, no. 1 (2022): 190, https://doi.org/10.3390/pharmaceutics14010190.

19. J. F. Lechner and G. D. Stoner, "Red Beetroot and Betalains as Cancer Chemopreventative Agents," *Molecules* 24, no. 8 (2019): 1602, https://doi.org/10.3390/molecules24081602.

20. Trinchieri et al., "Potential Renal Acid Load and the Risk of Renal Stone Formation in a Case-Control Study," *European Journal of Clinical Nutrition* 67, no. 10 (2013): 1077–80, https://doi.org/10.1038/ejcn.2013.155.

21. Eric N. Taylor and Gary C. Curhan, "Oxalate Intake and the Risk for Nephrolithiasis," *Journal of the American Society of Nephrology* 18, no. 7 (2007): 2198–2204, https://doi.org/10.1681/asn.2007020219.

22. Claudia D'Alessandro et al., "Which Diet for Calcium Stone Patients: A Real-World Approach to Preventive Care," *Nutrients* 11, no. 5 (2019): 1182, https://doi.org/10.3390/nu11051182.

23. Cupisti et al., "Insulin Resistance and Low Urinary Citrate Excretion in Calcium Stone Formers," *Biomedicine and Pharmacotherapy* 61, no. 1 (2007): 86–90, https://doi.org/10.1016/j.biopha.2006.09.012.

24. S. Joshi and D. S. Goldfarb, "The Use of Antibiotics and Risk of Kidney Stones," *Current Opinion in Nephrology and Hypertension* 28, no. 4 (2019): 311–5, https://doi.org/10.1097/MNH.0000000000000510.

25. Spiller et al, "Anti-Inflammatory Effects of Red Pepper (*Capsicum baccatum*) on Carrageenan- and Antigen-Induced Inflammation," *Journal of Pharmacy and Pharmacology* 60 (2008): 473–8, https://doi.org/10.1211/jpp.60.4.0010.

26. Weston Petroski and Deanna M. Minich, "Is There Such a Thing as 'Anti-Nutrients'? A Narrative Review of Perceived Problematic Plant Compounds," *Nutrients* 12, no. 10 (2020): 2929, https://doi.org/10.3390/nu12102929.

27. Salma F. Ahmad Fuzi et al., "A 1-H Time Interval between a Meal Containing Iron and Consumption of Tea Attenuates the Inhibitory Effects on Iron Absorption: A Controlled Trial in a Cohort of Healthy UK Women Using a Stable Iron Isotope," *The American Journal of Clinical Nutrition* 106, no. 6 (2017): 1413–21, https://doi.org/10.3945/ajcn.117.161364.

28. M. S. Djurhuus et al., "Insulin Increases Renal Magnesium Excretion: A Possible Cause of Magnesium Depletion in Hyperinsulinaemic States," *Diabetic Medicine* 12, no. 8 (1995): 664–69, https://doi.org/10.1111/j.1464-5491.1995.tb00566.x.

29. Petroski and Minich, "Is There Such a Thing as 'Anti-Nutrients'? A Narrative Review of Perceived Problematic Plant Compounds?" *Nutrients* 12, no. 10 (2020): 2929, https://doi.org/10.3390/nu12102929.

30. A. Kapała, M. Szlendak, and E. Motacka, "The Anti-Cancer Activity of Lycopene: A Systematic Review of Human and Animal Studies," *Nutrients* 14, no. 23 (2022): 5152, https://doi.org/10.3390/nu14235152.

31. A. V. Rao and S. Agarwal, "Role of Antioxidant Lycopene in Cancer and Heart Disease," *Journal of the American College of Nutrition* 19, no. 5 (2000): 563–9, https://doi.org/10.1080/07315724.2000.10718953.

32. Yao et al., "Quercetin, Inflammation and Immunity," *Nutrients* 8, no. 3 (2016): 167, https://doi.org/10.3390/nu8030167.

33. Schmelzer et al., "Functions of Coenzyme Q10 in Inflammation and Gene Expression," *BioFactors* 32 (2008): 179–83, https://doi.org/10.1002/biof.5520320121.

34. Najafi et al., "Effects of Alpha Lipoic Acid on Metabolic Syndrome: A Comprehensive Review," *Phytotherapy Research* 36, no 6 (2022): 2300–23, https://doi.org/10.1002/ptr.7406.

35. M. Eggersdorfer and A. Wyss, "Carotenoids in Human Nutrition and Health," *Archives of Biochemistry and Biophysics* 652 (2018): 18–26, https://doi.org/10.1016/j.abb.2018.06.001.

36. J. Pizzorno, "Glutathione!" *Integrative Medicine (Encinitas)* 13, no. 1 (2014): 8-12, https://www.ncbi.nlm.nih.gov/pmc/articles/PMC4684116/.

37. C. Perricone, C. De Carolis, and R. Perricone, "Glutathione: a Key Player in Autoimmunity," *Autoimmunity Reviews* 8, no. 8 (2009): 697–701, https://doi.org/10.1016/j.autrev.2009.02.020.

38. Dentico et al., "Il glutatione nella terapia delle epatopatie croniche steatosiche [Glutathione in the Treatment of Chronic Fatty Liver Diseases]." *Recenti progressi in medicina* 86 no. 7-8 (1995): 290-3, https://pubmed.ncbi.nlm.nih.gov/7569285/.

39. Rose et al., "Evidence of Oxidative Damage and Inflammation Associated with Low Glutathione Redox Status in the Autism Brain," *Translational Psychiatry* 2, no. 7 (2012): e134, https://doi.org/10.1038/tp.2012.61.

40. Tříska et al., "Factors Influencing Sulforaphane Content in Broccoli Sprouts and Subsequent Sulforaphane Extraction," *Foods* 10, no. 8 (2021): 1927, https://doi.org/10.3390/foods10081927.

41. H. Gill and G. Walker, "Selenium, Immune Function and Resistance to Viral Infections," *Nutrition and Dietetics* 65 (2008): S41-7, https://doi.org/10.1111/j.1747-0080.2008.00260.x.

42. M. Ventura , M. Melo, and F. Carrilho, "Selenium and Thyroid Disease: From Pathophysiology to Treatment," *International Journal of Endocrinology* (2017): 1297658, https://doi.org/10.1155/2017/1297658.

43. Fritz et al., "Selenium and Lung Cancer: A Systematic Review and Meta Analysis," *PLOS One* (2011), https://doi.org/10.1371/journal.pone.0026259.

44. M. P. Rayman, "The Importance of Selenium to Human Health," *The Lancet* 356, no. 9225 (2000): 233–41, https://doi.org/10.1016/S0140-6736(00)02490-9.

45. A. Chauhan and V. Chauhan, "Beneficial Effects of Walnuts on Cognition and Brain Health," *Nutrients* 12, no. 2 (2020): 550, https://doi.org/10.3390/nu12020550.

46. Guasch-Ferré et al., "Effects of Walnut Consumption on Blood Lipids and Other Cardiovascular Risk Factors: an Updated Meta-Analysis and Systematic Review of Controlled Trials," *The American Journal of Clinical Nutrition* 108, no. 1 (2018): 174-87, https://doi.org/10.1093/ajcn/nqy091.

47. Yang et al., "Walnut Intake May Increase Circulating Adiponectin and Leptin Levels but Does Not Improve Glycemic Biomarkers: A Systematic Review and Meta-Analysis of Randomized Clinical Trials," *Complementary Therapies in Medicine* 52 (2020): 102505, https://doi.org/10.1016/j.ctim.2020.102505.

48. A. Magnussen and M. A. Parsi, "Aflatoxins, Hepatocellular Carcinoma and Public Health," *World Journal of Gastroenterology* 19, no. 10 (2013): 1508–12, https://doi.org/10.3748/wjg.v19.i10.1508.

49. B. Y. Silber and J. A. J. Schmitt, "Effects of Tryptophan Loading on Human Cognition, Mood, and Sleep," *Neuroscience and Biobehavioral Reviews* 34, no. 3 (2010): 387-407, https://doi.org/10.1016/j.neubiorev.2009.08.005.

50. Buck et al., "Meta-Analyses of Lignans and Enterolignans in Relation to Breast Cancer Risk," *The American Journal of Clinical Nutrition* 92, no. 1 (2010): 141–53, https://doi.org/10.3945/ajcn.2009.28573.

51. Ogawa et al., "Sesame Lignans Modulate Cholesterol Metabolism in the Stroke-Prone Spontaneously Hypertensive Rat," *Clinical and Experimental Pharmacology and Physiology* 22 (1995): S310-2, https://doi.org /10.1111/j.1440-1681.1995.tb02932.x.

52. Peterson et al., "Dietary Lignans: Physiology and Potential for Cardiovascular Disease Risk Reduction," *Nutrition Reviews* 68, no. 10 (2010): 571–603, https://doi.org/10.1111/j.1753-4887.2010.00319.x.

53. Gillian Flower et al., "Flax and Breast Cancer: A Systematic Review," *Integrative Cancer Therapies* 13, no. 3 (2013): 181–92, https://doi.org/10.1177/ 1534735413502076.

54. Keys et al., "The Diet and 15-Year Death Rate in the Seven Countries Study," *American Journal of Epidemiology* 124, no. 6 (1986): 903–15, https://doi.org /10.1093/oxfordjournals.aje.a114480.

55. Chowdhury et al., "Association of Dietary, Circulating, and Supplement Fatty Acids with Coronary Risk: a Systematic Review and Meta-Analysis," *Annals of Internal Medicine* 160, no. 6 (2014): 398–406, https://doi.org/10.7326 /M13-1788.

56. Siri-Tarino et al., "Meta-Analysis of Prospective Cohort Studies Evaluating the Association of Saturated Fat with Cardiovascular Disease," *The American Journal of Clinical Nutrition* 91, no. 3 (2010): 535–46, https://doi.org.10.3945/ ajcn.2009.27725.

57. Harcombe et al., "Evidence from Randomised Controlled Trials Did Not Support the Introduction of Dietary Fat Guidelines in 1977 and 1983: A Systematic Review and Meta-Analysis," *Open Heart* 2, no. 1 (2015): e000196, https://doi.org/10.1136/openhrt-2014-000196.

58. Petursson et al., "Is the Use of Cholesterol in Mortality Risk Algorithms in Clinical Guidelines Valid? Ten Years Prospective Data from the Norwegian HUNT 2 Study," *Journal of Evaluation in Clinical Practice* 18, no. 1 (2012): 159–68, https://doi.org/10.1111/j.1365-2753.2011.01767.x.

59. G. A. Soliman, "Dietary Cholesterol and the Lack of Evidence in Cardiovascular Disease," *Nutrients* 10, no. 6 (2018): 780, https://doi.org/10.3390/ nu10060780.

60. P. J. Jones, "Dietary Cholesterol and the Risk of Cardiovascular Disease in Patients: A Review of the Harvard Egg Study and Other Data," *International Journal of Clinical Practice, Supplement* 163 (2009): 1–8, 28–36, https://doi.org /10.1111/j.1742-1241.2009.02136.x.

61. Berger et al., "Dietary Cholesterol and Cardiovascular Disease: A Systematic Review and Meta-Analysis," *The American Journal of Clinical Nutrition* 102, no. 2 (2015): 276–94, https://doi.org/10.3945/ajcn.114.100305.

62. Babak Bagheri et al., "The Ratio of Unesterified/Esterified Cholesterol Is the Major Determinant of Atherogenicity of Lipoprotein Fractions," *Medical Archives* 72, no. 2 (2018): 103, https://doi.org/10.5455/medarh.2018.72.103-107.

63. Danaei et al., "The Preventable Causes of Death in the United States: Comparative Risk Assessment of Dietary, Lifestyle, and Metabolic Risk Factors," *PLoS Medicine* 6, no. 4 (2009): e1000058, https://doi.org/10.1371/journal.pmed.1000058.

64. Susan Hewlings, "Coconuts and Health: Different Chain Lengths of Saturated Fats Require Different Consideration," *Journal of Cardiovascular Development and Disease* 7, no. 4 (December 17, 2020): 59, https://doi.org/10.3390/jcdd7040059.

65. Khaw et al., "Randomised Trial of Coconut Oil, Olive Oil or Butter on Blood Lipids and Other Cardiovascular Risk Factors in Healthy Men and Women," *BMJ Open* 8, no. 3 (2018): e020167, https://doi.org/10.1136/bmjopen-2017-020167.

66. S. Intahphuak, P. Khonsung, and A. Panthong, "Anti-Inflammatory, Analgesic, and Antipyretic Activities of Virgin Coconut Oil," *Pharmaceutical Biology* 48, no. 2 (2010): 151-7, https://doi.org/10.3109/13880200903062614.

67. Nitbani et al., "Antimicrobial Properties of Lauric Acid and Monolaurin in Virgin Coconut Oil: A Review," *ChemBioEng Reviews* 9 (2022): 442-61, https://doi.org/10.1002/cben.202100050.

68. Febri Odel Nitbani et al., "Antimicrobial Properties of Lauric Acid and Monolaurin in Virgin Coconut Oil: A Review," *ChemBioEng Reviews* 9, no. 5 (2022): 442-61, https://doi.org/10.1002/cben.202100050.

69. Boateng et al. "Coconut Oil and Palm Oil's Role in Nutrition, Health and National Development: A Review," *Ghana Medical Journal* 50, no. 3 (2016): 189-96, https://www.ncbi.nlm.nih.gov/pmc/articles/PMC5044790/.

70. P. Sandupama, D. Munasinghe, and M. Jayasinghe, "Coconut Oil as a Therapeutic Treatment for Alzheimer's Disease: A Review," *Journal of Future Foods* 2, no. 1 (2022): 41-52, https://doi.org/10.1016/j.jfutfo.2022.03.016.

71. Usharani et al., "Effect of NCB-02, Atorvastatin and Placebo on Endothelial Function, Oxidative Stress and Inflammatory Markers in Patients with Type 2 Diabetes Mellitus: A Randomized, Parallel-Group, Placebo-Controlled, 8-Week Study," *Drugs in R&D* 9, no. 4 (2008): 243-50, https://doi.org/10.2165/00126839-200809040-00004.

72. Lal et al., "Efficacy of Curcumin in the Management of Chronic Anterior Uveitis," *Phytotherapy Research* 13, no. 4 (1999): 318-22, https://doi.org/10.1002/(SICI)1099-1573(199906)13:4<318::AID-PTR445>3.0.CO;2-7.

73. Takada et al., "Nonsteroidal Anti-Inflammatory Agents Differ in Their Ability to Suppress NF-kappaB Activation, Inhibition of Expression of Cyclooxygenase-2 and Cyclin D1, and Abrogation of Tumor Cell Proliferation," *Oncogene* 23, no. 57 (2004): 9247-58, https://doi.org/10.1038/sj.onc.1208169.

74. R. B. van Breemen, Y. Tao, and W. Li, "Cyclooxygenase-2 Inhibitors in Ginger (*Zingiber officinale*)," *Fitoterapia* 82, no. 1 (2011), 38–43, https://doi.org /10.1016/j.fitote.2010.09.004.

75. Kalt et al., "Recent Research on the Health Benefits of Blueberries and Their Anthocyanins," *Advances in Nutrition* 11, no. 2 (2020): 224-236, https://doi.org /10.1093/advances/nmz065.

76. Rodriguez-Mateos et al., "Circulating Anthocyanin Metabolites Mediate Vascular Benefits of Blueberries: Insights From Randomized Controlled Trials, Metabolomics, and Nutrigenomics," *The Journals of Gerontology: Series A* 74, no. 7 (2019): 967-976, https://doi.org/10.1093/gerona/glz047.

Chapter 5

1. J. J. DiNicolantonio, J. H. O'Keefe, and W. L. Wilson, "Sugar Addiction: Is It Real? A Narrative Review," *British Journal of Sports Medicine* 52 (2018): 910-3, https://bjsm.bmj.com/content/52/14/910.

2. "Sugar Consumption by Country," World Population Review, https://world populationreview.com/country-rankings/sugar-consumption-by-country.

3. "Added Sugars," American Heart Association, https://www.heart.org/en/ healthy-living/healthy-eating/eat-smart/sugar/added-sugars#:~:text=For%20 most%20American%20women%2C%20that's,day%2C%20or%20about%20 9%20teaspoons.).

4. P. Moreira, "High-Sugar Diets, Type 2 Diabetes and Alzheimer's Disease," *Current Opinion in Clinical Nutrition and Metabolic Care* 16, no. 4 (2013): 440-5, https://doi.org/10.1097/MCO.0b013e328361c7d1.

5. G. A. Bray and B. M. Popkin, "Dietary Sugar and Body Weight: Have We Reached a Crisis in the Epidemic of Obesity and Diabetes?: Health Be Damned! Pour on the Sugar," *Diabetes Care* 37, no. 4 (2014): 950-6, https:// doi.org/10.2337/dc13-2085.

6. Huang et al., "Sugar Sweetened Beverages Consumption and Risk of Coronary Heart Disease: A Meta-Analysis of Prospective Studies," *Atherosclerosis* 234, no. 1 (2014): 11-6, https://doi.org/10.1016/j.atherosclerosis.2014.01.037.

7. Debras et al., "Total and Added Sugar Intakes, Sugar Types, and Cancer Risk: Results from the Prospective NutriNet-Santé Cohort," *The American Journal of Clinical Nutrition* 112, no. 5 (2020): 1267-79, https://doi.org/10.1093/ ajcn/nqaa246.

8. Chen et al., "Consumption of Sugar-Sweetened Beverages Has a Dose-Dependent Effect on the Risk of Non-Alcoholic Fatty Liver Disease: An Updated Systematic Review and Dose-Response Meta-Analysis," *International Journal of Environmental Research and Public Health* 16, no. 12 (2019): 2192, https://doi.org/10.3390/ijerph16122192.

9. Miao et al., "Sugar in Beverage and the Risk of Incident Dementia, Alzheimer's Disease and Stroke: A Prospective Cohort Study," *The Journal of Prevention of Alzheimer's Disease* 8 (2021): 188-93, https://doi.org/10.14283/ jpad.2020.62.

10. Debras et al., "Artificial Sweeteners and Cancer Risk: Results from the Nutri-Net-Santé Population-Based Cohort Study," *PLOS Medicine* (2022), https://doi.org/10.1371/journal.pmed.1003950.

11. Fowler et al., "Fueling the Obesity Epidemic? Artificially Sweetened Beverage Use and Long-Term Weight Gain," *Obesity (Silver Spring)* 16, no. 8 (2008): 1894–900, https://doi.org/10.1038/oby.2008.284.

12. Mathur et al., "Effect of Artificial Sweeteners on Insulin Resistance among Type-2 Diabetes Mellitus Patients," *Journal of Family Medicine and Primary Care* 9, no. 1 (2020): 69–71, https://doi.org/10.4103/jfmpc.jfmpc_329_19.

13. Debras et al., "Artificial Sweeteners and Risk of Cardiovascular Diseases: Results from the Prospective NutriNet-Santé Cohort," *The BMJ* 378 (2022): e071204, https://doi.org/10.1136/bmj-2022-071204.

14. Witkowski et al., "The Artificial Sweetener Erythritol and Cardiovascular Event Risk," *Nature Medicine* 29 (2023): 710–718, https://doi.org/10.1038/s41591-023-02223-9.

15. Jackson et al., "Neurologic and Psychiatric Manifestations of Celiac Disease and Gluten Sensitivity," *Psychiatric Quarterly* 83, no. 1 (2012): 91–102, https://doi.org/10.1007/s11126-011-9186-y.

16. Behall et al., "Diets Containing High Amylose vs Amylopectin Starch: Effects on Metabolic Variables in Human Subjects," *The American Journal of Clinical Nutrition* 49, no. 2 (1989): 337–344, https://doi.org/10.1093/ajcn/49.2.337.

17. Vahdat et al. "Effects of Resistant Starch Interventions on Circulating Inflammatory Biomarkers: A Systematic Review and Meta-Analysis of Randomized Controlled Trials," *Nutrition Journal* 19, no. 33 (2020), https://doi.org/10.1186/s12937-020-00548-6.

18. M. Kasuga, "Insulin Resistance and Pancreatic Beta Cell Failure," *Journal of Clinical Investigation* 116, no. 7 (2006): 1756–60, https://doi.org/10.1172/JCI29189.

19. Vaziri et al., "High Amylose Resistant Starch Diet Ameliorates Oxidative Stress, Inflammation, and Progression of Chronic Kidney Disease," *PLoS One* (2014), https://doi.org/10.1371/journal.pone.0114881.

20. Kabir et al., "Dietary Amylose-Amylopectin Starch Content Affects Glucose and Lipid Metabolism in Adipocytes of Normal and Diabetic Rats," *The Journal of Nutrition* 128, no. 1 (1998): 35–42, https://doi.org/10.1093/jn/128.1.35.

21. S. E. Shoelson, J. Lee, and A. B. Goldfine, "Inflammation and Insulin Resistance," *Journal of Clinical Investigation* 116, no. 7 (2006): 1793–801, https://doi.org/10.1172/JCI29069.

22. James J. DiNicolantonio and James H. O'Keefe, "Low-Grade Metabolic Acidosis as a Driver of Insulin Resistance," *Open Heart* 8, no. 2 (2021): e001788, https://doi.org/10.1136/openhrt-2021-001788.

23. "Cancer: Carcinogenicity of the Consumption of Red Meat and Processed Meat," World Health Organization, https://www.who.int/news-room/questions-and-answers/item/cancer-carcinogenicity-of-the-consumption-of-red-meat-and-processed-meat.

24. S. Larsson and A. Wolk, "Red and Processed Meat Consumption and Risk of Pancreatic Cancer: Meta-Analysis of Prospective Studies," *British Journal of Cancer* 106 (2012): 603-7, https://doi.org/10.1038/bjc.2011.585.

25. R. Micha, G. Michas, and D. Mozaffarian, "Unprocessed Red and Processed Meats and Risk of Coronary Artery Disease and Type 2 Diabetes—An Updated Review of the Evidence," *Current Atherosclerosis Reports* 14 (2012): 515-24, https://doi.org/10.1007/s11883-012-0282-8.

26. Quan et al., "Association of Dietary Meat Consumption Habits with Neurodegenerative Cognitive Impairment: an Updated Systematic Review and Dose-Response Meta-Analysis of 24 Prospective Cohort Studies," *Food and Function* 24 (2022), https://doi.org/10.1039/D2FO03168J.

27. R. Micha, S. K. Wallace, and D. Mozaffarian, "Red and Processed Meat Consumption and Risk of Incident Coronary Heart Disease, Stroke, and Diabetes Mellitus: A Systematic Review and Meta-Analysis," *Circulation* 121, no. 21 (2010): 2271-83, https://doi.org/10.1161/CIRCULATIONAHA.109.924977.

28. "Cheese Accounts for Largest Share of Per Capita U.S. Dairy Product Consumption," USDA.gov, https://www.ers.usda.gov/data-products/chart-gallery/gallery/chart-detail/?chartId=103984#:~:text=Overall%20U.S.%20dairy%20consumption%20remained%20roughly%20the%20same%20over%20this,equivalents%20per%20person%20in%201979.

29. Chen et al., "Dairy Fat and Risk of Cardiovascular Disease in 3 Cohorts of US Adults," *The American Journal of Clinical Nutrition* 104, no. 5 (2016): 1209-17, https://doi.org/10.3945/ajcn.116.134460.

30. McCann et al., "Usual Consumption of Specific Dairy Foods Is Associated with Breast Cancer in the Roswell Park Cancer Institute Data Bank and BioRepository," *Current Developments in Nutrition* 1, no. 3 (2017): e000422, https://doi.org/10.3945/cdn.117.000422.

31. Aune et al., "Dairy Products, Calcium, and Prostate Cancer Risk: A Systematic Review and Meta-Analysis of Cohort Studies," *The American Journal of Clinical Nutrition* 101, no. 1 (2015): 87-117, https://doi.org/10.3945/ajcn.113.067157.

32. Lumia et al., "Food Consumption and Risk of Childhood Asthma," *Pediatric Allergy and Immunology* 26, no. 8 (2015): 789-96, https://doi.org/10.1111/pai.12352.

33. R. G. Cumming and R. J. Klineberg, "Case-Control Study of Risk Factors for Hip Fractures in the Elderly," *American Journal of Epidemiology* 139, no. 5 (1994): 493-503, https://doi.org/10.1093/oxfordjournals.aje.a117032.

34. Feskanich et al., "Milk, Dietary Calcium, and Bone Fractures in Women: A 12-Year Prospective Study," *American Journal of Public Health* 87, no. 6 (1997): 992-7, https://doi.org/10.2105/ajph.87.6.992.

35. Michaëlsson et al., "Milk Intake and Risk of Mortality and Fractures in Women and Men: Cohort Studies," *The BMJ* 349 (2014): g6015, https://doi.org/10.1136/bmj.g6015.

36. Na et al., "Association of Galactose and Insulin Resistance in Polycystic Ovary Syndrome: A Case-Control Study," *The Lancet* 47 (2022), https://doi.org/10.1016/j.eclinm.2022.101379.

37. Escrich et al., "Effects of Diets High in Corn Oil or in Extra Virgin Olive Oil on Oxidative Stress in an Experimental Model of Breast Cancer," *Molecular Biology Reports* 47, no. 7 (2020): 4923-32, https://doi.org/10.1007/s11033-020-05492-6.

38. J. J. DiNicolantonio and J. O'Keefe, "The Importance of Maintaining a Low Omega-6/Omega-3 Ratio for Reducing the Risk of Autoimmune Diseases, Asthma, and Allergies," *Missouri Medicine* 118, no. 5 (2021): 453-9, https://www.ncbi.nlm.nih.gov/pmc/articles/PMC8504498/.

39. Tsurutani et al., "Increased Serum Dihomo-γ-linolenic Acid Levels Are Associated with Obesity, Body Fat Accumulation, and Insulin Resistance in Japanese Patients with Type 2 Diabetes," *Internal Medicine* 57, no. 20 (2018): 2929-35, https://doi.org/10.2169/internalmedicine.0816-18.

40. Artemis P. Simopoulos, "The Importance of the Omega-6/Omega-3 Fatty Acid Ratio in Cardiovascular Disease and Other Chronic Diseases," *Experimental Biology and Medicine* 233, no. 6 (2008): 674-88, https://doi.org/10.3181/0711-mr-311.

41. Apte et al., "A Low Dietary Ratio of Omega-6 to Omega-3 Fatty Acids May Delay Progression of Prostate Cancer," *Nutrition and Cancer* 65, no. 4 (2013): 556-62, https://doi.org/10.1080/01635581.2013.775316.

42. Tsurutani et al., "Increased Serum Dihomo-γ-linolenic Acid Levels."

43. Blasbalg et al., "Changes in Consumption of Omega-3 and Omega-6 Fatty Acids in the United States during the 20th Century," *The American Journal of Clinical Nutrition* 93, no. 5 (2011): 950-62, https://doi.org/10.3945/ajcn.110.006643.

Chapter 6

1. Liwen Wang et al., "How Does the Tea L-Theanine Buffer Stress and Anxiety," *Food Science and Human Wellness* 11, no. 3 (2022): 467-75, https://doi.org/10.1016/j.fshw.2021.12.004.

2. Roger Highfield, "Chlorine in Water Increases Birth Defects," *Telegraph*, June 2, 2008, https://www.telegraph.co.uk/news/science/science-news/3343364/Chlorine-in-water-increases-birth-defects.html.

3. Kate Gibson, "Chemicals in Tap Water Could Cause 100,000 Cases of Cancer in U.S.," CBS News, https://www.cbsnews.com/news/chemicals-in-tap-water-could-cause-100000-cases-of-cancer-in-u-s/.

4. Jordanna Schriever, "Cancer Alert over South Australia's Tap Water," *Advertiser*, October 13, 2012, Sunday Mail, News section, https://www.adelaidenow.com.au/news/south-australia/cancer-alert-over-south-australias-tap-water/news-story/a6b7f393a40b0e0bb13aa3f24222e11a.

5. Ann Moore, "West Virginia Chemical Spill Triggers Tap Water Ban," Reuters, January 9, 2014, https://www.reuters.com/article/us-usa-westvirginia-spill-idUKBREA0902T20140110.

6. Douglas Main, "Brain-Eating Amoeba in Tap Water Killed Child, Study Confirms," *Newsweek*, January 25, 2015, Tech & Science section, https://www.newsweek.com/brain-eating-amoeba-tap-water-killed-child-study-confirms-301738.

7. Kayla Jimenez, "Lead in School Water Persists in US Despite Work to Fix the Problem. What Can Be Done?" *USA Today*, February 23, 2023 (Updated February 24, 2023), Education section, https://www.usatoday.com/story/news/education/2023/02/23/lead-persists-us-schools-despite-attempts-fix/11316247002/.

8. Gloria Odalipo, "Toxic Arsenic Levels Make Tap Water Unsafe for Thousands in New York City," *The Guardian*, September 6, 2022, US section, https://www.theguardian.com/us-news/2022/sep/06/toxic-arsenic-levels-tap-water-unsafe-nyc.

9. Johny Fernandez, "Dangerous Arsenic Levels Found in Tap Water at Manhattan NYCHA Complex," ABC 7 Eyewitness News, September 4, 2022, https://abc7ny.com/arsenic-nycha-jacob-riis-houses-water-in-wter/12196559/.

10. "State of American Drinking Water," EWG.org, https://www.ewg.org/tapwater/state-of-american-drinking-water.php.

Chapter 7

1. F. H. Nielsen, "Magnesium Deficiency and Increased Inflammation: Current Perspectives," *Journal of Inflammation Research* 11 (2018): 25–34, https://doi.org/10.2147/JIR.S136742.

2. Memarzia et al., "Experimental and Clinical Reports on Anti-Inflammatory, Antioxidant, and Immunomodulatory Effects of *Curcuma longa* and Curcumin, an Updated and Comprehensive review," *BioFactors* 47 (2021): 311–50, https://doi.org/10.1002/biof.1716.

3. V. P. Menon and A. R. Sudheer, "Antioxidant and Anti-Inflammatory Properties of Curcumin," in *The Molecular Targets and Therapeutic Uses of Curcumin in Health and Disease*, eds. B. B. Aggarwal, Y. J. Surh, and S. Shishodia (Boston: Springer, 2007), https://doi.org/10.1007/978-0-387-46401-5_3.

4. M. C. Fadus et al., "Curcumin: An Age-Old Anti-Inflammatory and Anti-Neoplastic Agent," *Journal of Traditional and Complementary Medicine* 7, no. 3 (2017): 339–46, https://doi.org/10.1016/j.jtcme.2016.08.002.

Chapter 8

1. Welch et al., "Urine pH Is an Indicator of Dietary Acid-Base Load, Fruit and Vegetables and Meat Intakes: Results from the European Prospective Investigation into Cancer and Nutrition (EPIC)-Norfolk Population Study," *British Journal of Nutrition* 99, no. 6 (2008): 1335–43, https://doi.org/10.1017/S0007114507862350.

Chapter 9

1. Anand et al., "Cancer is a Preventable Disease That Requires Major Lifestyle Changes," *Pharmaceutical Research* 25, no. 9 (2008): 2097-116, https://doi.org/10.1007/s11095-008-9661-9.

2. "Simple Steps to Preventing Diabetes," Harvard T.H. Chan School of Public Health (The Nutrition Source), https://www.hsph.harvard.edu/nutritionsource/disease-prevention/diabetes-prevention/preventing-diabetes-full-story/.

3. Howard LeWine, "200,000 Heart Disease, Stroke Deaths a Year Are Preventable," Harvard Health Blog, Harvard Medical School, September 4, 2013, https://www.health.harvard.edu/blog/200000-heart-disease-stroke-deaths-a-year-are-preventable-201309046648.

4. "Preventing Stroke: Healthy Living," Centers for Disease Control and Prevention and Health Promotion, January 2017. https://www.cdc.gov/stroke/prevention.htm

5. "Prevention and Risk of Alzheimer's and Dementia," Alzheimer's Association Research Center, 2018. https://www.alz.org/alzheimers-dementia/research_progress/prevention

6. T. Buclin et al., "Diet Acids and Alkalis Influence Calcium Retention in Bone," *Osteoporosis International* 12, no. 6 (2001): 493-99, https://doi.org/10.1007/s001980170095.

7. Bess Dawson-Hughes et al., "Treatment with Potassium Bicarbonate Lowers Calcium Excretion and Bone Resorption in Older Men and Women," *The Journal of Clinical Endocrinology & Metabolism* 94, no. 1 (2009): 96–102, https://doi.org/10.1210/jc.2008-1662.

8. Fatemeh Gholami et al., "The Association of Dietary Acid Load (DAL) with Estimated Skeletal Muscle Mass and Bone Mineral Content: A Cross-Sectional Study," *BMC Nutrition*, 9 (2023), https://doi.org/10.1186/s40795-022-00658-w.

9. H. Lambert et al., "The Effect of Supplementation with Alkaline Potassium Salts on Bone Metabolism: A Meta-Analysis," *Osteoporosis International* 26, no. 4 (2015): 1311–18, https://doi.org/10.1007/s00198-014-3006-9.

10. J. Negrete-Corona, J. C. Alvarado-Soriano, and L. A. Reyes-Santiago, "Fractura de cadera como factor de riesgo en la mortalidad en pacientes mayores de 65 años. Estudio de casos y controles [Hip Fracture as Risk Factor for Mortality in Patients over 65 Years of Age. Case-Control Study]," *Acta ortopédia Mexicana* 28, no. 6 (2014): 352–62, https://pubmed.ncbi.nlm.nih.gov/26016287/.

11. Dawson-Hughes et al., "Alkaline Diets Favor Lean Tissue Mass in Older Adults," *The American Journal of Clinical Nutrition* 87, no. 3 (2008): 662-5, https://doi.org/10.1093/ajcn/87.3.662.

12. Welch et al., "A Higher Alkaline Dietary Load Is Associated with Greater Indexes of Skeletal Muscle Mass in Women," *Osteoporosis International* 24 (2013): 1899–908, https://doi.org/10.1007/s00198-012-2203-7.

13. Alexy et al., "Long-Term Protein Intake and Dietary Potential Renal Acid Load Are Associated with Bone Modeling and Remodeling at the Proximal Radius in Healthy Children," *The American Journal of Clinical Nutrition* 82, no. 5 (2005): 1107-14, https://doi.org/10.1093/ajcn/82.5.1107.

14. Caciano et al., "Effects of Dietary Acid Load on Exercise Metabolism and Anaerobic Exercise Performance," *Journal of Sports Science and Medicine* 14, no. 2 (2015): 364-71, https://www.ncbi.nlm.nih.gov/pmc/articles/PMC4424466/.

15. Chycki et al., "Alkaline Water Improves Exercise-Induced Metabolic Acidosis and Enhances Anaerobic Exercise Performance in Combat Sport Athletes," *PLoS One* (2018), https://doi.org/10.1371/journal.pone.0205708.

16. Halz et al., "Beta-Alanine Supplementation and Anaerobic Performance in Highly Trained Judo Athletes," *Baltic Journal of Health and Physical Activity* 14, no. 2 (2022): Article 1, https://doi.org/10.29359/BJHPA.14.2.01.

17. Durkalec-Michalski et al., "The Effect of Beta-Alanine versus Alkaline Agent Supplementation Combined with Branched-Chain Amino Acids and Creatine Malate in Highly-Trained Sprinters and Endurance Athletes: A Randomized Double-Blind Crossover Study," *Nutrients* 11, no. 9 (2019): 1961, https://doi.org/10.3390/nu11091961.

Chapter 10

1. Fildes et al., "Probability of an Obese Person Attaining Normal Body Weight: Cohort Study Using Electronic Health Records," *American Journal of Public Health* 105, no. 9 (2015): e54-9, https://doi.org/10.2105/AJPH.2015.302773.

2. Gruzdeva et al., "Leptin Resistance: Underlying Mechanisms and Diagnosis," *Diabetes, Metabolic Syndrome and Obesity* 12 (2019): 191-8, https://doi.org/10.2147/DMSO.S182406.

3. Your basal metabolic rate (BMR) is *the number of calories your body requires to fulfill its most basic life-sustaining functions.* Average estimates are 2,000 for females and 2,500 for males.

4. A. G. Dulloo and J. Jacquet, "Adaptive Reduction in Basal Metabolic Rate in Response to Food Deprivation in Humans: A Role for Feedback Signals from Fat Stores," *The American Journal of Clinical Nutrition* 68, no. 3 (1998): 599-606, https://doi.org/10.1093/ajcn/68.3.599.

5. Sumithran et al., "Long-Term Persistence of Hormonal Adaptations to Weight Loss," *The New England Journal of Medicine* 365, no. 17 (2011): 1597-604, https://doi.org/10.1056/NEJMoa1105816.

6. M. E. Lean and D. Malkova, "Altered Gut and Adipose Tissue Hormones in Overweight and Obese Individuals: Cause or Consequence?" *International Journal of Obesity (London)* 40, no. 4 (2016): 622-32, https://doi.org/10.1038/ijo.2015.220.

Chapter 11

1. K. Beaudoin and D. S. Willoughby, "The Role of the Gluten-Derived Peptide Gliadin in Celiac Disease," *Journal of Nutritional Health and Food Engineering* 1, no. 6 (2014): 229–32, https://doi.org/10.15406/jnhfe.2014.01.00036.

2. Brand et al., "The Role of Mitochondrial Function and Cellular Bioenergetics in Ageing and Disease," *British Journal of Dermatology* 169, Suppl 2(0 2), (2013): 1–8, https://doi.org/10.1111/bjd.12208.

3. Putti et al., "Diet Impact on Mitochondrial Bioenergetics and Dynamics," *Frontiers in Physiology* 6 (2015), https://doi.org/10.3389/fphys.2015.00109.

4. Kyriazis et al., "The Impact of Diet upon Mitochondrial Physiology (Review)," *International Journal of Molecular Medicine* 50, no. 5 (2022): 135, https://doi.org/10.3892/ijmm.2022.5191.

5. Bikman et al., "A High-Carbohydrate Diet Lowers the Rate of Adipose Tissue Mitochondrial Respiration," *European Journal of Clinical Nutrition* 76 (2022): 1339–42, https://doi.org/10.1038/s41430-022-01097-3.

6. Peri-Okonny et al., "High-Phosphate Diet Induces Exercise Intolerance and Impairs Fatty Acid Metabolism in Mice," *Circulation* 139, no. 11 (2019): 1422–34, https://doi.org/10.1161/CIRCULATIONAHA.118.037550.

7. K. Niaz, E. Zaplatic, and J. Spoor, "Extensive Use of Monosodium Glutamate: A Threat to Public Health?" *EXCLI Journal* 17 (2018): 273–8, https://doi.org/10.17179/excli2018-1092.

8. P. Humphries, E. Pretorius, and H. Naudé, "Direct and Indirect Cellular Effects of Aspartame on the Brain," *European Journal of Clinical Nutrition* 62, 451–62 (2008), https://doi.org/10.1038/sj.ejcn.1602866.

9. Pase et al., "Sugar- and Artificially Sweetened Beverages and the Risks of Incident Stroke and Dementia: A Prospective Cohort Study," *Stroke* 48, no. 5 (2017): 1139–46, https://doi.org/10.1161/STROKEAHA.116.016027.

10. Van den Eeden et al., "Aspartame Ingestion and Headaches: A Randomized Crossover Trial," *Neurology* 44, no. 10 (1994): 1787–93, https://doi.org/10.1212/wnl.44.10.1787.

11. W. A. Klee, C. Zioudrou, and R. A. Streaty, "Exorphins: Peptides with Opioid Activity Isolated from Wheat Gluten, and Their Possible Role in the Etiology of Schizophrenia," in *Endorphins in Mental Health Research*, eds. E. Usdin, W. E. Bunney, and N. S. Kline (London: Palgrave Macmillan, 1979), https://doi.org/10.1007/978-1-349-04015-5_18.

12. I. F. Robey, "Examining the Relationship between Diet-Induced Acidosis and Cancer," *Nutrition and Metabolism (London)* 9, no. 72 (2012), https://doi.org/10.1186/1743-7075-9-72.

13. Lacourt et al., "The High Costs of Low-Grade Inflammation: Persistent Fatigue as a Consequence of Reduced Cellular-Energy Availability and Non-Adaptive Energy Expenditure," *Frontiers in Behavioral Neuroscience* 12 (2018): 78, https://doi.org/10.3389/fnbeh.2018.00078.

14. Akula et al., "Antifungal Efficacy of Lauric Acid and Caprylic Acid—Derivatives of Virgin Coconut Oil against Candida albicans," *Biomedical and Biotechnology Research Journal (BBRJ)* 5 (2021): 229-34, https://doi.org/10.4103/bbrj.bbrj_65_21.

Chapter 12

1. J. Appleton, "The Gut-Brain Axis: Influence of Microbiota on Mood and Mental Health," *Integrative Medicine (Encinitas)* 17, no. 4 (2018): 28-32, https://www.ncbi.nlm.nih.gov/pmc/articles/PMC6469458/.

2. Huang et al., "Current Understanding of Gut Microbiota in Mood Disorders: An Update of Human Studies," *Frontiers in Genetics* 10 (2019), 98, https://doi.org/10.3389/fgene.2019.00098.

3. Christina Maser, Sanziana Roman, and Arbjorn Toset, "Gastrointestinal Manifestations of Endocrine Disease," *World Journal of Gastroenterology* 12, no. 20 (2006): 3174-3179, https://doi.org/10.3748/wjg.v12.i20.3174.

Chapter 13

1. Berger et al., "Mediation of the Acute Stress Response by the Skeleton," *Cell Metabolism* 30, no. 5 (2019): 890-902.e8, https://doi.org/10.1016/j.cmet.2019.08.012.

2. L. Frassetto et al., "Diet, Evolution and Aging," *European Journal of Nutrition* 40, no. 5 (2001): 200-213, https://doi.org/10.1007/s394-001-8347-4.

3. Tanushree Banerjee, Anthony Sebastian, and Lynda Frassetto, "Association of Diet-Dependent Systemic Acid Load, Renal Function, and Serum Albumin Concentration," *Journal of Renal Nutrition* 33, no. 3 (2023): 428-434, https://doi.org/10.1053/j.jrn.2023.01.007.

4. C. Palacios, "The Role of Nutrients in Bone Health, from A to Z," *Critical Reviews in Food Science and Nutrition* 46, no. 8 (2006): 621-628, https://doi.org/10.1080/10408390500466174.

5. Feskanich et al., "Milk, Dietary Calcium, and Bone Fractures in Women: A 12-Year Prospective Study," *American Journal of Public Health* 87, no. 6 (1997): 992-7, https://doi.org/10.2105/ajph.87.6.992.

6. Feskanich et al., "Milk Consumption during Teenage Years and Risk of Hip Fractures in Older Adults," *JAMA Pediatrics* 168, no. 1 (2014): 54-60, https://doi.org/10.1001/jamapediatrics.2013.3821.

7. Lacey Bourassa, "Vegan and Plant-Based Diet Statistics for 2023," Plant Proteins.co, https://www.plantproteins.co/vegan-plant-based-diet-statistics/.

8. "Osteoporosis," Centers for Disease Control and Prevention (National Center for Health Statistics), https://www.cdc.gov/nchs/fastats/osteoporosis.htm.

9. M. Martyn-St James and S. Carroll, "Meta-Analysis of Walking for Preservation of Bone Mineral Density in Postmenopausal Women," *Bone* 43, no. 3 (2008): 521-31, https://doi.org/10.1016/j.bone.2008.05.012.

10. Filho et al., "Rebound Training Modifies Body Composition, Muscular Strength and Bone Health Indicators in Adult Women," *EC Endocrinology and Metabolic Research* 4.8 (2019): 326–335, https://www.researchgate.net/profile/Hugo-Filho-2/publication/336926983_Rebound_Training_Modifies_Body_Composition_Muscular_Strength_and_Bone_Health_Indicators_in_Adult_Women/links/5dbb31c8299bf1a47b0704c7/Rebound-Training-Modifies-Body-Composition-Muscular-Strength-and-Bone-Health-Indicators-in-Adult-Women.pdf.

Chapter 14

1. "General Information/Press Room," American Thyroid Association, https://www.thyroid.org/media-main/press-room.

2. "Thyroid—Hypothyroidism," Better Health Channel, https://www.betterhealth.vic.gov.au/health/conditionsandtreatments/thyroid-hypothyroidism.

3. Wyne et al., "Hypothyroidism Prevalence in the United States: A Retrospective Study Combining National Health and Nutrition Examination Survey and Claims Data, 2009-2019," *Journal of the Endocrine Society* 7, no. 1 (2023): bvac172, https://doi.org/10.1210/jendso/bvac172.

4. I. F. Robey, "Examining the Relationship between Diet-Induced Acidosis and Cancer," *Nutrition and Metabolism (London)* 9, no. 72 (2012), https://doi.org/10.1186/1743-7075-9-72.

5. M. Chu and T. F. Seltzer, "Myxedema Coma Induced by Ingestion of Raw Bok Choy," *The New England Journal of Medicine* 362, no. 20 (2010): 1945–6, https://doi.org/10.1056/NEJMc0911005.

6. Weston Petroski and Deanna M. Minich, "Is There Such a Thing as 'Anti-Nutrients'? A Narrative Review of Perceived Problematic Plant Compounds," *Nutrients* 12, no. 10 (2020): 2929, https://doi.org/10.3390/nu12102929.

7. M. Brüngger, H. N. Hulter, and R. Krapf, "Effect of Chronic Metabolic Acidosis on Thyroid Hormone Homeostasis in Humans," *American Journal of Physiology* 272, no. 5 (Pt 2), (1997): F648–53, https://doi.org/10.1152/ajprenal.1997.272.5.F648.

8. Luo et al., "Sleep Disturbance and Incidence of Thyroid Cancer in Postmenopausal Women The Women's Health Initiative," *American Journal of Epidemiology* 177, no. 1 (2013): 42–9, https://doi.org/10.1093/aje/kws193.

9. Choi et al., "Association between Obstructive Sleep Apnea and Thyroid Cancer Incidence: A National Health Insurance Data Study," *European Archives of Oto-Rhino-Laryngology* 278, no. 11 (2021): 4569–74, https://doi.org/10.1007/s00405-021-06896-1.

Chapter 15

1. Iddir et al., "Strengthening the Immune System and Reducing Inflammation and Oxidative Stress through Diet and Nutrition: Considerations during the COVID-19 Crisis," *Nutrients* 12, no. 6 (2020): 1562, https://doi.org/10.3390/nu12061562.

2. Kumar et al., "Physiopathology and Management of Gluten-Induced Celiac Disease," *Journal of Food Science* 82 (2017): 270-7, https://doi.org/10.1111/1750-3841.13612.

3. D. Sarkar, M. K. Jung, and H. J. Wang, "Alcohol and the Immune System," *Alcohol Research: Current Reviews* 37, no. 2 (2015): 153-5, https://www.ncbi.nlm.nih.gov/pmc/articles/PMC4590612/.

4. D. A. Ehwarieme, E. I. Odum, and O. O. Whiliki, "Effect of Nutritive and Non-Nutritive Sweeteners on Gut Microbiota of Healthy Adult Individuals," *Nigerian Journal of Science and Environment* 18, no. 1 (2022), https://delsunjse.com/index.php/njse/article/view/57.

5. Bischoff et al., "Possible Adverse Effects of Food Additive E171 (Titanium Dioxide) Related to Particle Specific Human Toxicity, Including the Immune System," *International Journal of Molecular Sciences* 22, no. 1 (2021): 207, https://doi.org/10.3390/ijms22010207.

6. Abou-Donia et al., "Splenda Alters Gut Microflora and Increases Intestinal P-Glycoprotein and Cytochrome P-450 in Male Rats," *Journal of Toxicology and Environmental Health, Part A* 71, no. 21 (2008): 1415-29, https://doi.org/10.1080/15287390802328630.

7. M. K. Hostetter, "Handicaps to Host Defense: Effects of Hyperglycemia on C3 and *Candida albicans*," *Diabetes* 39, no. 3 (1990): 271-5, https://doi.org/10.2337/diab.39.3.271.

8. P. Kubes and C. Jenne, "Immune Responses in the Liver," *Annual Review of Immunology* 36 (2018): 247-77, https://doi.org/10.1146/annurev-immunol-051116-052415.

9. Chassaing et al., "Dietary Emulsifiers Impact the Mouse Gut Microbiota Promoting Colitis and Metabolic Syndrome," *Nature* 519 (2015): 92-6, https://doi.org/10.1038/nature14232.

10. Hassan et al., "The Effects of Monosodium Glutamate on Thymic and Splenic Immune Functions and Role of Recovery (Biochemical and Histological study)," *Journal of Cytology and Histology* 5, no. 6 (2014): 1000283, https://doi.org/10.4172/2157-7099.1000283.

11. Vorland et al., "Effects of Excessive Dietary Phosphorus Intake on Bone Health," *Current Osteoporosis Reports* 15, no. 5 (2017): 473-82, https://doi.org/10.1007/s11914-017-0398-4.

12. Matthew J. Goodman, "The 'Natural' vs. 'Natural Flavors' Conflict in Food Labeling: A Regulatory Viewpoint," *Food and Drug Law Journal* 72 (2017): 78-102, https://pubmed.ncbi.nlm.nih.gov/29140655/.

13. Josh Bloom, "Natural and artificial flavors: What's the difference?," American Council on Science and Health, 2017, https://www.acsh.org/sites/default/files/Natural-and-Artificial-Flavors-What-s-the-Difference.pdf.

Chapter 16

1. "National Diabetes Statistics Report," Centers for Disease Control and Prevention, https://www.cdc.gov/diabetes/data/statistics-report/index.html

2. Igarashi et al., "Effect of Acidosis on Insulin Binding and Glucose Uptake in Isolated Rat Adipocytes," *The Tohoku Journal of Experimental Medicine* 169, no. 3 (1993): 205–13, https://doi.org/10.1620/tjem.

3. Esche et al., "Higher Diet-Dependent Renal Acid Load Associates with Higher Glucocorticoid Secretion and Potentially Bioactive Free Glucocorticoids in Healthy Children," *Kidney International* 90, no. 2 (2016): 325–333, https://doi.org/10.1016/j.kint.2016.02.033.

4. Kamba et al., "Association between Higher Serum Cortisol Levels and Decreased Insulin Secretion in a General Population," *PLoS One* 11, no. 11 (2016): e0166077, https://doi.org/10.1371/journal.pone.0166077.

5. Disthabanchong et al., "Metabolic Acidosis Lowers Circulating Adiponectin through Inhibition of Adiponectin Gene Transcription," *Nephrology Dialysis Transplantation* 26, no. 2 (2011): 592–8, https://doi.org/10.1093/ndt/gfq410.

6. K. W. Lee and D. Shin, "Positive Association between Dietary Acid Load and Future Insulin Resistance Risk: Findings from the Korean Genome and Epidemiology Study," *Nutrition Journal* 19, no. 137 (2020), https://doi.org/10.1186/s12937-020-00653-6.

7. Fagherazzi et al., "Dietary Acid Load and Risk of Type 2 Diabetes: The E3N-EPIC Cohort Study," *Diabetologia* 57 (2014): 313–20, https://doi.org/10.1007/s00125-013-3100-0.

8. G. M. Guest, B. Mackler, and H. C. Knowles, "Effects of Acidosis: Effects of Acidosis on Insulin Action and on Carbohydrate and Mineral Metabolism," *Diabetes* 1, no. 4 (1952): 276–82, https://doi.org/10.2337/diab.1.4.276.

Chapter 17

1. "Prevention," World Heart Federation, https://world-heart-federation.org/what-we-do/prevention/.

2. Howard LeWine, "200,000 Heart Disease, Stroke Deaths a Year Are Preventable," Harvard Health Blog, Harvard Medical School, September 4, 2013, https://www.health.harvard.edu/blog/200000-heart-disease-stroke-deaths-a-year-are-preventable-201309046648.

3. J. Ostrowska, J. Janiszewska, and D. Szostak-Węgierek, "Dietary Acid Load and Cardiometabolic Risk Factors-A Narrative Review," *Nutrients* 12, no. 11 (2020): 3419, https://doi.org/10.3390/nu12113419.

4. Akter et al., "High Dietary Acid Load Is Associated with Increased Prevalence of Hypertension: The Furukawa Nutrition and Health Study," *Nutrition* 31, no. 2 (2015): 298–303, https://doi.org/10.1016/j.nut.2014.07.007.

5. Parohan et al., "Dietary Acid Load and Risk of Hypertension: A Systematic Review and Dose-Response Meta-Analysis of Observational Studies," Nutrition, Metabolism and Cardiovascular Diseases 29, no. 7 (2019): 665–75, https://doi.org/10.1016/j.numecd.2019.03.009.

6. Park et al., "Association between the Markers of Metabolic Acid Load and Higher All-Cause and Cardiovascular Mortality in a General Population with Preserved Renal Function," *Hypertension Research* 38 (2015): 433–8, https://doi.org/10.1038/hr.2015.23.

7. Turusheva et al., "Low Cholesterol Levels Are Associated with a High Mortality Risk in Older Adults without Statins Therapy: An Externally Validated Cohort Study," *Archives of Gerontology and Geriatrics* 90 (2020): 104180, https://doi.org/10.1016/j.archger.2020.104180.

8. Nago et al., "Low Cholesterol Is Associated with Mortality from Stroke, Heart Disease, and Cancer: the Jichi Medical School Cohort Study," *Journal of Epidemiology* 21, no. 1 (2011): 67–74, https://doi.org/10.2188/jea.je20100065.

9. Lappe et al., "Vitamin D and Calcium Supplementation Reduces Cancer Risk: Results of a Randomized Trial," *The American Journal of Clinical Nutrition* 85, no. 6 (2007): 1586–91, https://doi.org/10.1093/ajcn/85.6.1586.

10. G. K. Schwalfenberg, "A Review of the Critical Role of Vitamin D in the Functioning of the Immune System and the Clinical Implications of Vitamin D Deficiency," *Molecular Nutrition and Food Research* 55 (2011): 96–108, https://doi.org/10.1002/mnfr.201000174.

11. De Martinis et al., "Vitamin D Deficiency, Osteoporosis and Effect on Autoimmune Diseases and Hematopoiesis: A Review," *International Journal of Molecular Sciences* 22, no. 16 (2021): 8855, https://doi.org/10.3390/ijms22168855.

12. A. D. Höck, "Vitamin D3 Deficiency Results in Dysfunctions of Immunity with Severe Fatigue and Depression in a Variety of Diseases," *In Vivo* 28, no. 1 (2014): 133–45, https://iv.iiarjournals.org/content/28/1/133.short.

13. Liu et al., "Long-Term Increase in Cholesterol Is Associated with Better Cognitive Function: Evidence from a Longitudinal Study," *Frontiers in Aging Neuroscience* 13 (2021): 691423, https://doi.org/10.3389/fnagi.2021.691423.

14. Svensson et al., "The Association between Midlife Serum High-Density Lipoprotein and Mild Cognitive Impairment and Dementia after 19 Years of Follow-Up," *Translational Psychiatry* 9, no. 26 (2019), https://doi.org/10.1038/s41398-018-0336-y.

15. Papakostas et al. "Cholesterol in Mood and Anxiety Disorders: Review of the Literature and New Hypotheses," *European Neuropsychopharmacology* 14, no. 2 (2004): 135–42, https://doi.org/10.1016/S0924-977X(03)00099-3.

16. G. A. Soliman, "Dietary Cholesterol and the Lack of Evidence in Cardio-vascular Disease," *Nutrients* 10, no. 6 (2018): 780, https://doi.org/10.3390/nu10060780.

17. Vergara et al., "Associations of Changes in Blood Lipid Concentrations with Changes in Dietary Cholesterol Intake in the Context of a Healthy Low-Carbohydrate Weight Loss Diet: A Secondary Analysis of the DIETFITS Trial," *Nutrients* 13, no. 6 (2021): 1935, https://doi.org/10.3390/nu13061935.

18. M. P. St-Onge and P. J. Jones, "Greater Rise in Fat Oxidation with Medium-Chain Triglyceride Consumption Relative to Long-Chain Triglyceride Is Associated with Lower Initial Body Weight and Greater Loss of Subcutaneous Adipose Tissue," *International Journal of Obesity and Related Metabolic Disorders* 27, no. 12 (2003): 1565–71, https://doi.org/10.1038/sj.ijo.0802467.

19. N. D. Shah and B. N. Limketkai, "The Use of Medium-Chain Triglycerides in Gastrointestinal Disorders," (2017), https://med.virginia.edu/ginutrition/wp-content/uploads/sites/199/2014/06/Parrish-February-17.pdf.

20. P. Schönfeld and L. Wojtczak, "Short- and Medium-Chain Fatty Acids in Energy Metabolism: the Cellular Perspective," *Journal of Lipid Research* 57, no. 6 (2016): 943–54, https://doi.org/10.1194/jlr.R067629.

21. Augustin et al., "Mechanisms of Action for the Medium-Chain Triglyceride Ketogenic Diet in Neurological and Metabolic Disorders," *The Lancet Neurology* 17, no. 1 (2018): 84–93, https://doi.org/10.1016/S1474-4422(17)30408-8.

22. Rasmussen et al., "Efficacy of Supplemental MCT Oil on Seizure Reduction of Adult Drug-Resistant Epilepsy—A Single-Center Open-Label Pilot Study," *Nutritional Neuroscience* 26, no. 6 (2023): 535–9, https://doi.org/10.1080/1028415X.2022.2065816.

23. F. Labarthe, R. Gélinas, and C. Des Rosiers, "Medium-Chain Fatty Acids as Metabolic Therapy in Cardiac Disease," *Cardiovascular Drugs and Therapy* 22 (2008): 97–106, https://doi.org/10.1007/s10557-008-6084-0.

24. K. Nagao and T. Yanagita, "Medium-Chain Fatty Acids: Functional Lipids for the Prevention and Treatment of the Metabolic Syndrome," *Pharmacological Research* 61, no. 3 (2010): 208–12, https://doi.org/10.1016/j.phrs.2009.11.007.

Chapter 18

1. "Take Control of Your Cancer Risk: Nearly Fifty Percent of Common Cancers Are Preventable," American Institute for Cancer Research, https://www.aicr.org/news/take-control-of-your-cancer-risk-nearly-fifty-percent-of-common-cancers-are-preventable/.

2. "Statistics on Preventable Cancers," Cancer Research UK, https://www.cancerresearchuk.org/health-professional/cancer-statistics/risk/preventable-cancers.

3. "Cancer," World Health Organization, https://www.who.int/health-topics/cancer#tab=tab_1.

4. "Preventable cancers," International Agency for Research on Cancer, https://cancerpreventioneurope.iarc.fr/preventable-cancers/.

5. Anand et al., "Cancer is a Preventable Disease That Requires Major Lifestyle Changes," *Pharmaceutical Research* 25, no. 9 (2008): 2097–116, https://doi.org/10.1007/s11095-008-9661-9.

6. O. Warburg, "The Metabolism of Carcinoma Cells," *The Journal of Cancer Research* 9, no. 1 (1925): 148–63, https://doi.org/10.1158/jcr.1925.148.

7. Park et al., "High Dietary Acid Load Is Associated with Risk of Breast Cancer: Findings from the Sister Study," *The FASEB Journal* 31, no. 51 (2017): 168.4, https://doi.org/10.1096/fasebj.31.1_supplement.168.4.

8. Jafari Nasab et al., "Diet-Dependent Acid Load and the Risk of Colorectal Cancer and Adenoma: a Case-Control Study," *Public Health Nutrition* 24, no. 14 (2021): 4474–81, https://doi.org/10.1017/S1368980020003420.

9. Ronco et al., "Dietary Acid Load and Bladder Cancer Risk: An Epidemiologic Case-Control Study," *Multidisciplinary Cancer Investigation* 6, no. 2 (2022): 1–12, https://doi.org/10.30699/mci.6.2.284-2.

10. Shi et al., "Dietary Acid Load and the Risk of Pancreatic Cancer: A Prospective Cohort Study," *Cancer Epidemiology, Biomarkers and Prevention* 30, no. 5 (2021): 1009–19, https://doi.org/10.1158/1055-9965.EPI-20-1293.

11. I. F. Robey, "Examining the Relationship between Diet-Induced Acidosis and Cancer," *Nutrition and Metabolism (London)* 9, no. 72 (2012), https://doi.org/10.1186/1743-7075-9-72.

Chapter 20

1. Baumeister et al., "Ego Depletion: Is the Active Self a Limited Resource?" *Journal of Personality and Social Psychology* 74, no. 5 (1998): 1252–65, https://doi.org/10.1037/0022-3514.74.5.1252.

Chapter 21

1. Chang et al., "Inadequate Hydration, BMI, and Obesity Among US Adults: NHANES 2009-2012," *The Annals of Family Medicine* 14, no. 4 (2016): 320–4, https://doi.org/10.1370/afm.1951.

2. Suhr et al., "The Relation of Hydration Status to Cognitive Performance in Healthy Older Adults," *International Journal of Psychophysiology* 53, no. 2 (2004): 121–5, https://doi.org/10.1016/j.ijpsycho.2004.03.003.

3. Radosavljević et al. "Fluid Intake and Bladder Cancer. A Case Control Study," *Neoplasma* 50, no. 3 (2003): 234–8, http://www.ncbi.nlm.nih.gov/pubmed/12937859.

4. Strippoli et al., "Fluid and nutrient Intake and Risk of Chronic Kidney Disease," *Nephrology (Carlton)* 16, no. 3 (2011): 326–34, https://doi.org/10.1111/j.1440-1797.2010.01415.x.

5. R. Siener and A. Hesse, "Fluid Intake and Epidemiology of Urolithiasis," *European Journal of Clinical Nutrition* 57, Suppl 2 (2003): S47-51, https://doi .org/10.1038/sj.ejcn.1601901.

6. Chan et al., "Water, Other Fluids, and Fatal Coronary Heart Disease: The Adventist Health Study," *American Journal of Epidemiology* 155, no. 9 (2002): 827-33, https://doi.org/10.1093/aje/155.9.827.

7. F. Manz and A. Wentz, "The Importance of Good Hydration for the Prevention of Chronic Diseases," *Nutrition Reviews* 63, suppl_1 (2005): S2-5, https:// doi.org/10.1111/j.1753-4887.2005.tb00150.x.

8. S. Hewlings, "Coconuts and Health: Different Chain Lengths of Saturated Fats Require Different Consideration," *Journal of Cardiovascular Development and Disease* 7, no. 4 (2020): 59, https://doi.org/10.3390/jcdd7040059.

9. "Food Irradiation | US EPA," United States Environmental Protection Agency, n.d., https://www.epa.gov/radtown/food-irradiation.

10. "Methyl Bromide," Public Health England, January 2019, https://assets .publishing.service.gov.uk/government/uploads/system/uploads/attachment _data/file/827821/Methyl_bromide_PHE_general_information_2019.pdf.

11. N. J. Dodd, "Free Radicals and Food Irradiation," *Biochemical Society Symposia* 61 (November 1, 1995): 247-58, https://doi.org/10.1042/bss0610247.

Chapter 22

1. A. W. C. Yuen, I. A. Walcutt, and J. W. Sander, "An Acidosis-Sparing Ketogenic (ASK) Diet to Improve Efficacy and Reduce Adverse Effects in the Treatment of Refractory Epilepsy," *Epilepsy and Behavior* 74 (2017): 15-21, https://doi.org/10.1016/j.yebeh.2017.05.032.

Chapter 24

1. Richard D. Mattes, "Hunger and Thirst: Issues in Measurement and Prediction of Eating and Drinking," *Physiology & Behavior* 100, no. 1 (2010): 22-32, https://doi.org/10.1016/j.physbeh.2009.12.026.

2. B. Wansink, J. E. Painter, and J. North, "Bottomless Bowls: Why Visual Cues of Portion Size May Influence Intake," *Obesity Research* 13, no. 1 (2005): 93-100, http://doi.org/10.1038/oby.2005.12.

3. J. E. Flood and B. J. Rolls, "Soup Preloads in a Variety of Forms Reduce Meal Energy Intake," *Appetite* 49, no. 3 (2007): 626-34, https://doi.org/10.1016/j .appet.2007.04.002.

4. Alexander Kokkinos et al., "Eating Slowly Increases the Postprandial Response of the Anorexigenic Gut Hormones, Peptide YY and Glucagon-like Peptide-1," *The Journal of Clinical Endocrinology & Metabolism* 95, no. 1 (2010): 333-37, https://doi.org/10.1210/jc.2009-1018.

Index

Acknowledgments

So many people have helped me get this out to the world, and I am eternally grateful to all of them.

First, of course, the deepest appreciation, gratitude, and thanks to my incredible publisher, Hay House, which is absolutely the best in the business. In particular, Lisa Cheng and Monica O'Connor. Your (at times brutal, ha!) honesty and your clarity and vision for this book made it so much more than I thought it could be. You invested yourselves in it as much as I did, and I will always be so grateful to you for that. It is always such a pleasure working with you. Thank you, thank you, thank you.

Thanks to the incredible art team at Hay House, led by the wonderful Tricia Breidenthal, who has brought the covers of both this book and *The Alkaline Reset Cleanse* to life.

And where would I be without Reid Tracy and Patty Gift, who started this whole journey for me? I would never have become an author without you and your trust in me. Thank you so much.

To my "Plat Group" family who have been with me for the entire "alkaline journey so far," with special thanks to Jeff Walker (literally none of this would have happened without your mentorship), John, Will, Stu, Bari, Blue, Michael, Olivier, Sebastien, David, Ruth, Susan, Lee, Ocean, Jon, Erico, Ryan, Michelle, Ellyn, Victor, Brian, Annie, Hallvard, Richard, Des, Farukh, Ricardo, David, and more!

Special thanks to the incredible scientists, researchers, and those in the lab who are continually bringing new learnings and evidence to light around how powerful this alkaline thing is! Lynda Frassetto, Joseph Pizzorno, Thomas Remer, Ian Robey, Caroline Passey, and more, thank you to all of you.

To my community! You are my people and you inspire me every day to keep going. So many of you have been here right from the beginning in the early 2000s, and I adore you all! Thank you for spreading the message, living alkaline, and inspiring those in your communities too.

A very special thanks and acknowledgment to Tony Robbins, Robert Young, and Joseph McClendon. Without that UPW 2003, I wouldn't be where I am today.

And thanks to the other health heroes out there who continue to inspire me, some of whom I consider my friends and others I one day hope to: Daryl Gioffre (love you, bro!), Kris Carr, Rhonda Patrick, Susan Peirce Thompson, Ty and Charlene Bollinger, Peter Attia, Sara Gottfried, Andrew Huberman, Matthew Walker, and so many more.

My incredible Mum and Dad, there is too much to say. I thank you for everything from the bottom of my heart: the entrepreneurial life you inspired me with and your understanding, support, and love through everything (and all of the challenges too). You are both an inspiration to me and shaped who I have become in so many ways. I love you so much.

And to my Australian family, Judy and Royston. Your home has been my safe place for so many years. Judy, you've given our family so much, I absolutely adore you and the family you created. Thank you so much for all the support and love. Royston, you are one of the biggest influences on me and have shaped how I see the world in so many ways. You taught me so much. I am so grateful for how you showed me to see positivity in everything, no matter what. I miss you every day.

And finally Tania, the love of my life. None of this would be possible without you. From your giving me the strength and confidence to go for this wild journey to your amazing support through the toughest of times, you are the most incredible person I have ever met. I am so grateful to have you in my life. The way you think and the questions you ask have led to us having the most incredible life, and I love that you continue to push me out of my comfort zone on a *very* regular basis. I could not possibly love you more.

And finally my boys! Leo, Joe, and Kai. You bring so much joy to my life and inspire me to strive to be the best person I can be. You teach me something new every day. I am so proud of you all.

About the Author

Ross Bridgeford is the author of *The Alkaline Reset Cleanse*. His programs, including The Alkaline Life Club, Alkaline Reset Cleanse Coaching Program, The Anti-Inflammation Breakthrough, as well as his Alkaline Recipe Book Series, have helped hundreds of thousands of people reach the health of their dreams.

He has been teaching and coaching people to achieve their biggest health, energy, and body goals for 20 years, and he knows how to keep it simple and make it easy, effortless, and delicious.

He lives in Brisbane, Australia, with his partner, Tania, their three children, and their dog, Millie.

Visit him online at **www.rossbridgeford.com**.

Hay House Titles of Related Interest

YOU CAN HEAL YOUR LIFE, the movie,
starring Louise Hay & Friends
(available as an online streaming video)
www.hayhouse.com/louise-movie

THE SHIFT, the movie,
starring Dr. Wayne W. Dyer
(available as an online streaming video)
www.hayhouse.com/the-shift-movie

* * *

*BEYOND LONGEVITY: A Proven Plan for Healing Faster,
Feeling Better, and Thriving at Any Age*, by Jason Prall

*CHRIS BEAT CANCER: A Comprehensive Plan for Healing
Naturally*, by Chris Wark

*FOOD MATTERS COOKBOOK: A Simple Gluten-Free Guide
to Transforming Your Health One Meal at a Time*,
by James Colquhoun and Laurentine ten Bosch

*REAL SUPERFOODS: Everyday Ingredients to
Elevate Your Health*,
by Ocean Robbins and Nichole Dandrea-Russert, MS, RDN

* * *

*All of the above are available at your local bookstore,
or may be ordered by visiting:*

Hay House USA: www.hayhouse.com®
Hay House Australia: www.hayhouse.com.au
Hay House UK: www.hayhouse.co.uk
Hay House India: www.hayhouse.co.in